A Practitioner's Guide to Telemental Health

A Practitioner's Guide to Telemental Health

How to Conduct Legal, Ethical, and Evidence-Based Telepractice

DAVID D. LUXTON, EVE-LYNN NELSON, and MARLENE M. MAHEU

American Psychological Association • Washington, DC

Published by
American Psychological Association
750 First Street, NE
Washington, DC 20002
www.apa.org

To order
APA Order Department
P.O. Box 92984
Washington, DC 20090-2984
Tel: (800) 374-2721; Direct: (202) 336-5510
Fax: (202) 336-5502; TDD/TTY: (202) 336-6123
Online: www.apa.org/pubs/books
E-mail: order@apa.org

In the U.K., Europe, Africa, and the Middle East, copies may be ordered from
American Psychological Association
3 Henrietta Street
Covent Garden, London
WC2E 8LU England

Typeset in Minion by Circle Graphics, Inc., Columbia, MD

Printer: Gasch Printing, Odenton, MD
Cover Designer: Mercury Publishing Services, Rockville, MD

Library of Congress Cataloging-in-Publication Data

Names: Luxton, David D., author. | Nelson, Eve-Lynn, author. | Maheu, Marlene M., author.
Title: A practitioner's guide to telemental health : how to conduct legal, ethical, and evidence-based telepractice / David D. Luxton, Eve-Lynn Nelson, Marlene M. Maheu.
Description: First edition. | Washington, DC : American Psychological Association, [2016] | Includes bibliographical references and index.
Identifiers: LCCN 2015050796| ISBN 9781433822278 | ISBN 143382227X
Subjects: LCSH: Medical telematics. | Telecommunication in medicine. | Mental health services.
Classification: LCC R119.95 .L89 2016 | DDC 610.285–dc23 LC record available at http://lccn.loc.gov/2015050796

British Library Cataloguing-in-Publication Data
A CIP record is available from the British Library.

Printed in the United States of America
First Edition

http://dx.doi.org/10.1037/14938-000

We dedicate this guidebook to the practitioner who is willing to change traditional methods of caring for those who struggle with behavioral and mental health challenges.

Contents

Foreword—Exciting Times

Patrick H. DeLeon, Omni Cassidy,
Joanna R. Sells, and Jane J. Abanes

With the enactment of President Obama's Patient Protection and Affordable Care Act (ACA) [P.L. 111-148], the United States has determined at the highest public policy level that all Americans will eventually have access to quality health care. The Congressional Budget Office estimated that by 2022, this legislation will provide an additional 33 million citizens with health insurance coverage, citizens who otherwise would have remained uninsured. The enactment of comprehensive health care reform has been a political quest for nearly every U.S. president since Franklin D. Roosevelt. Fundamental to the ACA is the development of the foundation for a significant transformation of our nation's health care system and the redefinition of "quality" health care.

Over the next decade, significant financial and structural incentives will be provided targeting the critical health policy goal of accomplishing "the triple aim"—that is, improving the experience of care, improving the health of populations, and reducing the cost of health care. As a nation, we have continued to spend more on health care than any other industrialized nation without achieving comparable health care outcomes. And numerous health policy experts have proposed that our continued history of unfortunate health disparities requires a comprehensive public health

The views expressed are those of the authors and do not reflect the official policy or position of the Uniformed Services University of the Health Sciences, the Department of Defense, or the U.S. Government.

approach involving community-based organizations and stakeholders if progress is ever to be realized. Telehealth provides a unique opportunity to reach those who otherwise would experience seemingly insurmountable barriers to accessing care.

In 2014, a little more than a decade after former President George W. Bush signed an Executive Order (#13335) establishing the position of national health information technology coordinator within the Department of Health and Human Services, coordinator Karen DeSalvo issued her *Federal Health IT Strategic Plan: 2015–2020*, identifying the federal government's health IT priorities, including those for telehealth technology. The report noted that since 2011, the health IT ecosystem has changed, with innovation occurring in mobile health applications and other technologies. The first goal enumerated was to accelerate the adoption and use of meaningful health IT (including telehealth and mobile health), with behavioral health being expressly identified. In her plan, one proposed strategy is to encourage the adoption of telehealth and mobile health technologies among providers and individuals, focusing on federal funding and/or programs providing health care and payment innovation model initiatives. This would include increasing access to broadband connectivity, especially in rural areas for health IT applications, such as high-resolution imaging, telehealth, and mobile health, as well as reforming payment systems to accommodate virtual care and telehealth. The underlying federal objective is to improve access to and the quality of health care services.

Internationally, progress with telemental health development is advancing rapidly. In 2010, the World Health Organization published a report titled *Telemedicine: Opportunities and Developments in Member States* to document the players and their projects. In the United States, professional associations in the behavioral disciplines began establishing standards and promulgating guidelines in the late 1990s and early 2000s. In 1999, Donna Ford, the American Counseling Association President, demonstrated bold leadership with a "cyber counseling committee" designed to develop standards for counselors working on the Internet. One of the authors of this guidebook, Marlene M. Maheu, served on that committee from 1999 to 2001. In 2008, the National Association of Social Workers published its guidelines. In 2009 and 2013, three American Telemedicine

Association (ATA) guidelines associated with telemental health were published. All three of the current guidebook's authors participated in the ATA work group related to the 2013 effort. The American Psychological Association published similar guidelines in 2013, under the leadership of then-President Melba Vasquez.

All of these efforts systematically addressed complex issues surrounding the delivery of behavioral care via technology—many of which are condensed and applied in this guidebook. For example, what is the scientific and clinical evidence regarding whether the overall quality of care differs as a function of the treatment modality and under what conditions? And, of course, how should interjurisdictional practice best be addressed?

Health care professionals must gain the necessary skills to conduct effective telemental health. The following text by Luxton, Nelson, and Maheu is a step-by-step guidebook for professionals to conduct telemental health care that is ethical and effective. The chapters in this volume underscore best practices, integration of technology, informed consent guidelines, ways to conduct assessments, and concerns regarding reliability and safety. The book also incorporates considerations for the needs of special clinics, including those in rural or underserved areas and serving specific groups. As we move into a new era of health care that uses critical technologies, this guidebook will be a mainstay in providing up-to-date information on effective delivery.

Acknowledgments

We are grateful to all who have engaged with us over the years and helped us to better understand the topics reflected in this guidebook. We appreciate the students who have trained with us for their ability to voice questions that expose the plain realities of "why, where, when, and how" to use technology in the practice of behavioral health care. We also acknowledge the dedication of our colleagues in academia, professional associations, the military, government offices, and regulatory boards as well as the information technologists, health care administrators, insurance company executives, communication specialists, economists, business developers, and entrepreneurs with whom we have consulted. We also acknowledge the pivotal role of the Coalition for Technology in Behavioral Science (CTiBS.org), the nonprofit organization forged to serve as a liaison between the national and international professional associations across behavioral health to advance the legal and ethical use of technology. We must also acknowledge the lifeblood of our work, our clients and patients. Their yearning for a better life has kept us awake, focused, and energized to meet their needs and serve them with the technologies of the 21st century.

We also wish to thank Linda Malnasi McCarter from APA Books for her steadfast support, guidance, and insistence that this telemental health guidebook is needed. We are grateful to Pat DeLeon for his vision and for showing us the importance of reaching beyond our professional borders to all behavioral disciplines. We thank Omni Cassidy, Joanna R. Sells, and Jane J. Abanes for their cogent contributions to our foreword, and we are grateful to Larry D. Pruitt, who provided feedback on an early draft of this guidebook. We are also grateful for the support of our families, whose understanding and patience humble us.

A Practitioner's Guide to Telemental Health

Introduction

The capability to provide behavioral health services with telecommunications technologies has greatly expanded avenues for behavioral and mental health professionals to provide quality care. This capability, which can be referred to as *telemental health* (TMH), has already extended to virtually all aspects of behavioral health service including the delivery of treatment, assessment, psychoeducation, supervision, and consultation. TMH has been used with almost every behavioral health diagnosis and across all age groups. The wide availability of desktop webcams, secure videoconferencing (VC) software, and improved high-speed networks can enable affordable access to care through traditional hospital, clinic, and office-based referrals or directly to the patient's home. Other technologies available to behavioral health providers that can be used to assist the TMH provider and augment care include mobile

http://dx.doi.org/10.1037/14938-001
A Practitioner's Guide to Telemental Health: How to Conduct Legal, Ethical, and Evidence-Based Telepractice, by D. D. Luxton, E.-L. Nelson, and M. M. Maheu

device health apps and interactive websites (Luxton, McCann, Bush, Mishkind, & Reger, 2011; Maheu, Pulier, & Roy, 2013; Mohr, Burns, Schueller, Clarke, & Klinkman, 2013).

To use any one of these technologies as a professional, however, requires competence and therefore appropriate training that includes competencies specific to the service delivered. Many of the issues associated with competent practice parallel those of conventional in-office services. However, professionals must extend competencies associated with existing skills practiced in traditional settings and also develop new skills that bridge the gaps created by geographical distance. For instance, a clinician may already be competent in suicide risk assessment and intervention. When practicing via VC, the clinician must complete a proper intake and assessment despite test instruments and procedures developed for in-office administration, continue to establish informed consent, obtain client/patient's emergency contact(s), involve emergency or support services if necessary at the client/patient's location, document essential elements of the procedure, and conduct appropriate follow-up at a distance. The physical distance between the clinician and the client/patient as well as the use of technology can create challenges, all of which are manageable when following best practices. For example, it is easy to hand out consent forms or administer paper-and-pencil assessments when in person, but additional steps are required when communicating by electronic mediums.

Just as with in-person services, TMH professionals need to know how to conduct practice consistent with the ethical standards, guidelines, and recommendations that are applicable to both their specific profession and the needs of their patient populations. Each discipline also has its own general ethics standards and sometimes guidelines, as established by the prevailing professional association(s). Some organizations have produced guidelines specific to telehealth practice. It is also necessary to know what legal requirements and liability risks are associated with TMH practice. Providers must ascertain whether TMH services are allowed to be provided and understand the unique accreditation, licensure, legal requirements, and advertising guidelines of the jurisdiction where the client/patient is located. The use of telehealth technologies also can present liability, even with the briefest of contact (e.g., e-mail, text message). Practitioners must be aware of intra- and interagency policies, including guidance on what and how particular services should be provided and the limits of those services. Another "need-to-know" requirement is informed consent, which must address patient safety, mandatory reporting requirements (e.g., duty to report with suicidal or homicidal clients/patients; mandated reporting of abuse to minors, elders, or partners), as well as privacy and data security.

In today's rapidly evolving technological landscape, practitioners need to be aware of which technologies are available, how to select the appropriate technologies, and how to optimize them for use. Telepractitioners also need to be sensitive to issues in clinically unsupervised settings—settings without clinical staff on-site, such as when care is provided directly to a client/patient who is located in his or her home at the time of the contact. Furthermore, TMH psychological assessment requires particular attention to factors that may influence the reliability, validity, and integrity of assessments and measures conducted remotely (e.g., unbeknownst to the professional, a family member may be present during part or all of the assessment procedure; clients/patients can easily look up answers to test questions while online; some assessments may be taken over the course of a week rather than at a single sitting).

Behavioral health services that are provided via technology also create a different context for the therapeutic process, including unique benefits and challenges. For example, telepractice extends the reach of service to underserved groups and diverse population that may have had limited previous contact with behavioral health services and/or with technology. Thus, it is crucial for clinicians to be familiar with how to work with clients/patients from diverse backgrounds. There are also potential complications that can arise during telepractice. For example, the clinician facing a delicate mandated reporting situation must be aware that an emotionally charged conversation with a client/patient about potential abuse may be more difficult to manage via VC. Such a client/patient may easily and quickly respond to abuse-related inquiries by simply turning off the computer. Such clients/patients are then unlikely to respond to attempts for further contact. Working via technology, then, also requires an understanding of how technology alters a professional clinical relationship and how to compensate for such alterations. Without proper training, clinicians may unwittingly put clients/patients and themselves at risk by treading into new terrain without full understanding and appreciation of these telepractice issues.

In recognizing the need to provide specific guidance, various professional associations in the behavioral sciences have developed ethical standards and/or guidelines for telepractice. Standards and guidelines help move TMH forward by increasing practitioner confidence and setting minimal standards for ethical and competent practice. They provide necessary high-level guidance but often lack the level of detail or practical recommendations needed by behavioral health practitioners. For this reason, TMH trainees and practitioners can benefit from a practice-friendly "how-to" guidebook that provides recommendations for conducting telepractice. In this book, we draw not only from relevant legal and regulatory codes, ethical standards, and guidelines but also from scientific literature and the hundreds of model TMH programs in the field.

Our purpose with this book, then, is to provide an essential how-to guide for conducting competent, ethical, and evidence-based TMH. In this guidebook, we focus primarily on the unique benefits and challenges of delivering real-time psychological services with VC equipment. Although we recognize that telephone, e-mail, text messaging, and other forms of communication technologies are used in practice (American Psychological Association, 2010b), we focus primarily on VC to give the interested clinician a quick yet broad-based overview of how to proceed with this particular modality. The researcher, educator, or practitioner who is interested in these other telehealth modalities is encouraged to see our list of resources available at the companion website: http://pubs.apa.org/books/supp/luxton/.

In the following pages, we outline best practices for establishing and conducting TMH services across diverse settings.

In Chapter 1, we introduce key definitions, the scope of TMH, and an overview of the benefits of TMH.

In Chapter 2, the reader will find an overview of currently available telehealth technologies with a focus on VC technologies and supporting software. This chapter also includes an overview of technologies that can be used to augment VC-based TMH (e.g., mHealth apps and other emerging technologies).

Chapter 3 describes legal, regulatory, and ethical issues in telepractice in public and private practice settings. The informed consent process is addressed, including compliance with various federal and state requirements related to telepractice. Privacy and data security issues are also discussed.

Chapter 4 walks the reader through the practical steps needed to establish a thriving TMH practice. Needs assessment and other administrative processes are outlined to help identify problem areas and key resources before engaging with clients/patients. Other topics addressed in this chapter include necessary documentation procedures.

Chapter 5 outlines how to develop safety plans for TMH services provided to clinically supervised (e.g., to a setting with trained support staff) as well as to unsupervised settings (e.g., to the homes of clients/patients). Topics include assessment of the appropriateness of TMH, emergency protocols, roles and responsibilities during emergency management, and risk management.

Full attention is given to the process of initiating and conducting TMH clinical sessions in Chapter 6. Best practices for establishing and maintaining therapeutic rapport are provided, including creating a welcoming telepractice environment. We share advice concerning best positioning of VC equipment (e.g., eye gaze) and troubleshooting technical problems. Special considerations are offered for conducting in-home TMH, as well as guidance for integrating other technologies (e.g., behavioral health apps).

Chapter 7 summarizes methods to ensure reliable and valid psychological assessments and testing conducted via telehealth technologies. We discuss selecting appropriate measures/tests, assuring optimal assessment conditions and procedures when using telehealth technologies, and delivering assessment results remotely.

Chapter 8 provides information on supervision and consultation services via telehealth technologies. We summarize the evidence base supporting remote supervision and teleconsultation, giving examples across a wide variety of trainees (e.g., predoctoral, postdoctoral, continuing education) and training settings.

In Chapter 9, we summarize strategies to promote clinical competency and multicultural sensitivity with diverse groups across the lifespan. We describe telepractice's potential to connect experts in working with specific populations (e.g., expertise with lesbian, gay, bisexual, transgender, queer, and intersex populations; expertise with rare medical disorders) with individuals seeking such behavioral and mental health services. A patient-centered approach is emphasized, taking into consideration how cultural factors and the broader community may influence the telepractice encounter and sustainable TMH service.

We conclude in Chapter 10 with summaries of issues discussed and descriptions of options and opportunities for practitioners interested in telepractice.

This guidebook is written for the new telepractitioner who wants to get started, the seasoned practitioner who seeks to continue to enhance TMH practice, the supervisor who engages in telesupervision, and the clinical manager or administrator interested in training a clinical team. The guidebook's practical recommendations also apply to TMH providers regardless of discipline or theoretical orientation. For our health professional (e.g., medicine, nursing, allied health) colleagues in areas beyond the traditional application of TMH in telepsychology, we have made conscious attempts to be inclusive of the broader health care arena across prevention and the behavioral components of chronic illness, including behavioral medicine, integrative medicine, and health psychology perspectives in many of our recommendations. Also, although this guidebook primarily uses examples of regulatory requirements and guidelines from the United States, it is also intended for the international behavioral and mental health researcher and practitioner communities.

TMH is a prospering area of practice that is expected to grow substantially in the years ahead. There is an expanding empirical literature base that supports its clinical effectiveness, including overall user acceptability and satisfaction among both clients/patients and care providers. In addition, public and private insurers are increasingly supporting the use of and reimbursement for some telehealth-based services. The capability to conduct behavioral services via telecommunications technologies has provided behavioral health professionals with opportunities to serve more people, specialize in areas of greatest professional development and interest, decrease office expense, and enjoy a mobile lifestyle from anywhere on the planet.

1

Concepts, Principles, and Benefits of Telemental Health

Telemental health has evolved from a rich history and variety of terms as different groups have sought to name their versions of behavioral and mental health care delivered across geographical distances (Maheu, Pulier, Wilhelm, McMenamin, & Brown-Connolly, 2004). Such terms include *telepsychiatry, telepsychology, behavioral telehealth, telebehavioral health, distance counseling, online therapy, e-therapy, web psychology, Internet therapy, teletherapy*, among others. For the purposes of this guidebook, we use *telemental health* or TMH as an umbrella term to refer to all of the names and types of behavioral and mental health services that are provided via telecommunications technologies. We use the phrases *TMH practitioners* and *telepractitioners* to refer to professionals engaged in the practice of either clinical or nonclinical aspects of health care provided via communications technology.

http://dx.doi.org/10.1037/14938-002
A Practitioner's Guide to Telemental Health: How to Conduct Legal, Ethical, and Evidence-Based Telepractice, by D. D. Luxton, E.-L. Nelson, and M. M. Maheu

Other noteworthy terms associated with TMH are *eHealth, remote monitoring*, and *mHealth.* eHealth refers to the use of the Internet to provide services, although this term is sometimes used more broadly to include other forms of technology. Web-based delivery of services, Internet chat, texting, and online social media are examples of such technologies. Remote monitoring refers to the growing field of monitoring vital signs and symptom report across geographic distance. Examples include heart rate, blood pressure, pulse, oxygen saturation levels, and blood glucose for a wide variety of chronic medical conditions, such as diabetes and hypertension. Mobile health, or the shortened mHealth, is the term used to describe health content or services that are provided on mobile devices such as smartphones and tablet devices (e.g., iPads). Software applications, or apps, are programs that operate on mobile devices.

VIDEOCONFERENCING AND TREATMENT SITES

Videoconferencing (VC) allows the clinician to converse with a client/patient and observe nonverbal behavior in real time. The visual component of VC creates a social presence that promotes familiarity, connectedness, and comfort for discussing complex topics that approximates the interactions of in-office settings. The ability to approximate on-site sessions led the Centers for Medicare and Medicaid Services (CMS) and other insurers in the United States to reimburse VC services in specified supervised settings (see http://www.cms.gov/telehealth).

Most laws and regulations in the United States define the site of care delivery where the client/patient is located as the *originating site*, which may be a remote clinic, a community center, or a residence. The clinician's site is most often referred to as the *distant site.* Another model to differentiate one site from another involves the hub-and-spoke model, which refers to the *spoke* as the client/patient's location, and the *hub* as the clinician's location (Maheu & McMenamin, 2004). We use the term *clinically supervised* to refer to locations that have clinical staff at the care delivery site. *Unsupervised* locations include the homes of clients/patients or other locations that may not have clinical staff on-site.

SCOPE OF TELEMENTAL HEALTH

TMH encompasses the entire gamut of clinical and administrative activities. These include behavioral or mental health treatment, substance use counseling, behavioral medicine, consumer or client/patient education (including the development and dissemination of self-help), and professional education.

The clinical uses of TMH are as extensive as those used in conventional in-person settings. Clinical TMH services may include

- clinical interviews for mental status, evaluation, diagnostics, and forensic evaluation;
- psychological testing, interpretation of results, and delivery of treatment recommendations;
- live treatment or intervention via VC;
- transmission of health data/assessment data (i.e., remote monitoring);
- clinical supervision; and
- clinical consultation and case management.

Nonclinical TMH applications include

- practice management, including recordkeeping, billing, scheduling, and transfer of materials (e.g., testing materials);
- distance education (for clients/patients or clinicians), which may include web-based discussion forums and chat rooms;
- administrative uses, including meetings among telehealth networks and presentations; and
- research and quality improvement.

TMH services are used in a wide range of settings, including hospitals and emergency departments, private practitioner offices, outpatient clinics, rehabilitation and other specialty hospitals, community mental health offices, and community health centers. Services may also be delivered in educational and other sites where services are needed (e.g., universities, schools, child-care centers, nursing homes, correctional facilities, churches, and corporate settings). Other settings may include oil rigs, ships, the battlefield, a hotel room, a library, the homes of clients/patients, or anywhere else the client/patient and clinician agree that it is appropriate to receive and deliver care.

There are practically no limits to where TMH can be implemented, as long as the services comply with applicable national, state, institutional, and professional regulations and policies. Telehealth-based services can also be combined with in-person services, as might be found by behavioral specialists who go to the home for in-person assessment and test administration, then deliver follow-up care with VC. The practice of TMH, however, does not remove any existing responsibilities in delivering services, such as adherence to the clinician's professional association codes of ethics, and state and federal laws (e.g., licensure, Health Insurance Portability and Accountability Act of 1996 [HIPAA]). In fact, it is the professional's responsibility to know and adhere to all applicable mandates and best practices, whichever technology the clinician chooses to use in the delivery of his or her professional services (Maheu, Pulier, McMenamin, & Posen, 2012).

BENEFITS OF TELEMENTAL HEALTH

The availability and capabilities of telepractice provide numerous benefits to providers and clients/patients alike. Depending on the circumstance, these overlapping benefits broadly include

- improved access to services and specialty services,
- decreased stigma (improved privacy that promotes willingness to seek care)
- clinical benefits (improved client/patient outcomes),
- convenience (time saving), and
- economic benefits (cost savings).

The gap between supply and demand for behavioral health services and the growing need for cost-effective services to reach more people is driving TMH's rapid expansion. Parity of general health and mental health services has also increased behavioral health coverage for some consumers, yet provider shortages continue to be a treatment barrier (Cunningham, 2009). An estimated 61.5 million Americans aged 18 and older experience some form of mental illness in a given year (National Institute of Mental

Health, n.d.), and about 9.2 million adults have co-occurring mental health and addiction disorders (U.S. Department of Health and Human Services, Substance Abuse and Mental Health Services Administration, Center for Behavioral Health Statistics and Quality, 2012). Furthermore, about 50% of adolescents aged 13 to 18 have experienced at least one mental health disorder in their lifetime (Merikangas et al., 2010). The majority of adults and children with behavioral health needs do not receive any services, let alone evidence-based assessment and treatment from trained mental health professionals. The gap between need and behavioral intervention is driven in part by a misdistribution of patients and providers (American Psychological Association, 2014), with gaps in rural areas as well as other underserved communities and populations. It is in part driven by absolute shortages in mental health providers, particularly in specialty areas.

TMH improves access to services for clients/patients living in geographically remote or medically underserved locations. According to the Health Resources and Services Administration (2014), approximately 80 million Americans live in a health professional shortage area (HPSA). These access gaps have remained or worsened as many rural communities have experienced shrinking populations, declining economies, and increasing poverty, as well as delays to treatment, less access to mental health insurance, and limited transportation options (Smalley, Warren, & Rainer, 2012).

Additional barriers prevent rural individuals from presenting to in-person clinics, including confidentiality concerns when one lives in a small community (Larson & Corrigan, 2010; Nelson & Bui, 2010). TMH addresses some of these concerns by offering access to a therapist outside of the community in nontraditional mental health settings that may be less stigmatizing, such as when visiting general health clinics, schools, and churches or perhaps directly in the home. VC approaches have also been successful in urban areas because of many of the same access concerns, particularly for underserved populations who may not be familiar with mental health services (Spaulding, Cain, & Sonnenschein, 2011), those who cannot easily traverse the complicated transit systems in cities, those who feel intimidated navigating the large health center environment, those experiencing homelessness, or those who have too many competing responsibilities to prioritize their behavioral and mental health needs over other economic and family pressures.

The use of TMH can also provide access to professionals in specialty areas (e.g., neuropsychological assessments). Moreover, TMH can connect clients/patients to professionals who have experience working with particular cultural groups (e.g., military culture, elderly persons, specific ethnic groups). TMH has the potential to increase communication across systems of care, including capabilities to link multiple individuals across multiple care systems. For example, with school-based telepractice, there is the opportunity for the child, parent(s), therapist, and school personnel to work together, enhancing both diagnosis and treatment.

TMH also provides unique clinical benefits to clients/patients that may result in improved treatment outcomes. For example, some clients/patients may feel less inhibited and, thus, more comfortable if they have the option to receive care in the comfort of their own home (Pruitt, Luxton, & Shore, 2014). There is anecdotal evidence that some adolescents prefer the increased personal space and control of their environment through technology (Nelson & Bui, 2010). Telehealth-based services may also facilitate connection with clients/patients who may otherwise lack social interaction, such as the client/patient who lives alone with limited social supports. It also allows clients/patients to stay closer to their local support network (family and friends) and involve those people in care (Maheu et al., 2004).

TMH may also promote patient-centered care and increase overall convenience. Hours of service can be extended, and technology can make it easier to follow up with clients/patients or provide check-ins between in-office visits or treatment sessions with brief visits that may last for 5 or 10 minutes. TMH may also provide the benefit of increasing continuity of care in between on-site visits, such as by allowing practitioners to conveniently monitor symptoms and patient "homework"/skill building activities. Moreover, the involvement of family members in helping with technology, safety planning, and other aspects of client/patient care may also facilitate a collaborative and supportive treatment environment that may have clinical benefits (Pruitt, Luxton, & Shore,

2014). Finally, telehealth technologies have the potential to facilitate integrated care consistent with the patient-centered medical home concept that provides clients/patients with highly coordinated and accessible patient-centered care.

Advantages also exist for the practitioner. TMH provides access to specific professionals and expert consultants that are not available in the local area. Some clinicians appreciate the conveniences of being able to serve more populations without needing to travel to other neighborhoods, cities, states, and even countries. Others appreciate the ability to move to distant states for retirement, yet continue serving the populations they have served during more active periods of their lives.

Telehealth-based services may provide several other economic benefits for both clients/patients and care providers. For one, clients/patients often experience fewer costs using telehealth (e.g., travel expenses and lost wages). TMH may decrease the need to pay for child care or eldercare when leaving the home for visits to a provider in another part of the state. Savings also can be related to the ability to avoid extended travel with dependents when caring for children with behavioral difficulties, as well as stresses navigating an unfamiliar health care setting and city.

Cost savings for care providers include reduced need for office space (i.e., a virtual practice). Group practices may benefit from reduced overall costs in sharing telehealth equipment and infrastructure, and telehealth provides the capability to share resources with and between clinical staff, such as supervision and consultation. Telehealth may also facilitate efficiency of tertiary care. That is, it can be used to identify clients/patients who may need more intensive care remotely and make recommendation for such care, if needed, without the expense of transport for conventional in-person assessment.

In the short term, TMH can increase costs or shift costs (Luxton, 2013). For example, setting up and sustaining a telepractice entails equipment and infrastructure costs. Fortunately, the ever-decreasing cost of technologies makes TMH more feasible and accessible than ever before. In the United States, health care reform has increased the appeal of using health information technologies through laws such as the Affordable Care

Act (Weinstein et al., 2014) and through increased parity in the coverage of telemedicine services across states (Thomas & Capistrant, 2015).

In summary, telepractice provides both opportunities and challenges. Professionals can now serve more people, specialize in areas of greatest interest, decrease office expenses, and enjoy a mobile lifestyle from anywhere on the planet—but they must be competent. They must understand the nuances of clinical care delivered from a distance; know how to operate the technology they select; and be in full compliance with legal, regulatory, and ethical requirements. Such competencies have been demonstrated in a wide variety of settings and are now outlined in this succinct how-to guide.

2

Overview of Telemental Health Technologies

Telemental health (TMH) practitioners must familiarize themselves with specific telehealth technologies, apply them appropriately, and understand risks and benefits to mitigate problems. This technical understanding is also essential as they educate their clients/patients about such issues as part of the informed consent process. Although the chapter focuses primarily on descriptions of technologies and how they are used in TMH, the reader is encouraged to review Chapter 3 for additional information regarding the privacy and data security, as well as technology-related information in the informed consent agreement.

http://dx.doi.org/10.1037/14938-003
A Practitioner's Guide to Telemental Health: How to Conduct Legal, Ethical, and Evidence-Based Telepractice, by D. D. Luxton, E.-L. Nelson, and M. M. Maheu

COMMUNICATION TYPES: SYNCHRONOUS VERSUS ASYNCHRONOUS

There are two primary categories of telehealth technologies: *synchronous* and *asynchronous.* Synchronous refers to live, real-time interactive two-way communication. Connections can occur between two or more parties simultaneously; videoconferencing (VC) and telephone are examples of synchronous communication modalities.

Asynchronous communication, also referred to as *store and forward,* is when information or data are collected and later sent to another location via electronic communication. This is often used when the clinician does not need to interact directly or in real time with the client/patient. An example of asynchronous communication is a substance abuse counselor conducting an assessment in accordance with a specific protocol in a rural area. The session could be videotaped and forwarded to a psychiatrist for review, treatment planning, and prescription of medication when needed and appropriate. These treatment recommendations are then forwarded to the substance abuse counselor or primary care or other prescribing professional at the originating site, where the patient is located. Other examples of asynchronous telecommunication technology include the secure e-mailing of consent and intake forms, clinical questionnaires, or surveys to clients/patients, as well as asking patients to go to a website to download such documents. Following institutional protocols, the client/patient can then be asked to fax paperwork to an office or scan it and upload it to a secured server with appropriate software. One-way text messaging services can also be used asynchronously to gather outcome data. With careful attention to security, other examples include faxing, scanning, or digital submission between the patient and provider sites to facilitate administrative functions.

Hybrid applications include combinations of synchronous, asynchronous, and/or in-person services. For example, following in-office clinical assessments, VC and telephone may be used for direct service from a clinician's office to a client/patient at home, and secure e-mail or mobile health apps can be used to send and retrieve forms.

VIDEOCONFERENCING

VC is the most common form of technology used for TMH. An advantage of VC versus telephone is that it more closely resembles the natural social experience of interacting with clients/patients. The video component of VC also allows TMH practitioners to observe and respond to nonverbal aspects interactions, such as eye contact and body movement. It also most closely resembles the training experiences given to clinicians who assess and/or diagnose and treat patients on-site. Another advantage of VC is that it helps TMH practitioners to more easily verify the identity of clients/patients (assuming they have previously identified them in person or by comparison through VC to enlarged driver's licenses or other photo identification). Importantly, VC services are often reimbursable when conducted in accordance with Medicare, Medicaid, and third-party carrier requirements. On the other hand, the use of the telephone is most often not reimbursable, typically because telephone encounters are usually viewed as brief and less similar to on-site services than are VC sessions. For more information about telehealth reimbursement, visit the federally funded resource center, the Center for Connected Health Policy (http://cchpca.org/), and the Center for Telehealth and e-Health Law (http://ctel.org/expertise/reimbursement/).

All VC systems consist of a camera for video, a microphone for audio, and a video monitor. These features are already present in many laptops and mobile devices, but specialized equipment may be desirable for the practitioner who wants to see the client/patient clearly while avoiding eyestrain. VC can also make use of high-end, dedicated equipment from manufacturers such as Cisco/Tandberg, LifeSize, and Polycom, among others. Which features are most suitable will depend on needs and costs. The use of personal computers and off-the-shelf webcams for Internet-based VC is an affordable and highly accessible option for home-based TMH. Most VC takes place via digital telephone lines (ISDN) or over a local area network (LAN), wide area network (WAN), or broadband Internet connection. Before panic sets in, the reader may want to know that most of the privacy and security requirements for any technology to be used in clinical care can be easily addressed by purchasing technology and related connectivity services through reputable vendors who give Business Associate Agreements (see Chapter 3, this volume).

Regardless of the type of VC equipment used, the technology should meet patient privacy and data security requirements consistent with applicable local guidelines. In the United States, for example, requirements are specified in the Health Insurance Portability and Accountability Act (HIPAA). Not to be neglected are the sometimes more stringent state-based requirements that must be followed (see Chapter 3).

When low bandwidth (slow Internet) is a problem, a tried-and-true solution involves the use of videophones. Low-bandwidth videophones are often found in situations or areas where higher bandwidth connections are either unavailable or too expensive. Two videophones connect to each other via traditional telephone lines, otherwise known as *plain old telephone service.* They look and operate much like telephones, using a telephone dial pad rather than a mouse to connect users to one another. Although videophones are inexpensive, they now face a declining market because of limited capability compared with other available technologies (e.g., cellular phones, free video apps that don't require downloading or executing files). Nonetheless, videophones are used in specific circumstances where their limited functionality is preferable to computers, such as in some nursing homes where elderly patients prefer them because of their familiarity with telephones or in prisons where the ability to connect to the Internet is undesirable.

FEATURES TO CONSIDER WITH VIDEOCONFERENCING

Specialized features exist to augment basic VC technology (e.g., recording capabilities; a camera that can pan, tilt, and zoom; picture-in-picture or PIP functionality to simultaneously view both the patient's and one's own image). Some VC software packages also allow for displaying computer files and programs, which can be useful for sharing documents with clients/patients, such as during clinical assessment or as part of psychoeducation. VC can also be augmented with the use of an electronic whiteboard, which allows users on both ends to share text and draw images or diagrams during a videoconferenced session. Internet relay chat and instant messaging are other features that allow users to send and receive text messages during VC. Many newer video platforms allow clients/patients to schedule sessions from their desktops with calendaring programs. An integrated calendaring system may also be useful to clinicians who do their own scheduling or to groups who wish to reduce scheduling staff expenses. Some larger video systems allow VC sessions to be embedded into their calendars, so clients and professionals alike can simply go to their calendars and click the date/time of the appointment; the VC software launches the session after a password is entered.

Some systems provide an opportunity for clients/patients to wait in a virtual waiting room, decorated with colors and furniture of their choice. Such newer features allow professionals to make a digital practice manageable, as well as creating the type of experience they prefer for the people they serve. Other systems allow for access to electronic health records (EHRs), professional training, practice management software, secured cloud storage, and much more.

Many vendors offer free trial periods. Take advantage of these to put in a few solid hours testing new platforms with colleagues. Be sure to review vendor offerings carefully and compare notes with a community of other clinicians who are also testing platforms before making a purchase, as well as refer to resources through professional organizations, training programs, and telehealth resource centers. This attention to essential operational skills will not only develop comfort and flexibility with the interface but will also help identify skill deficits prior to delivering professional care to potentially vulnerable patients.

TELEPHONE (VOICE-ONLY SYSTEMS)

The standard telephone for voice-only communication is another common medium used for telemental health. Basic telephone services are commonly used for scheduling and follow-up with clients/patients; they may also be used for psychological assessments when voice only is appropriate (Luxton, Pruitt, & Osenbach, 2014). For example, in some settings it may be appropriate to assess the status of patients (e.g., their mood, medication use) over the phone, but it may not be appropriate to conduct diagnostic assessment (for more information, see Chapter 7). Telephones also provide a reliable backup system to VC systems. Telephonic strategies have been shown to be effective in treating a range of conditions, including depression (Mohr, Vella, Hart, Heckman, & Simon, 2008). Some studies have shown that the telephone is preferable to specific groups of patients, such as African American dementia caregivers with depression (Glueckauf et al., 2012), and teleproviders are encouraged to seek information from their target population about technology preferences. Obviously, this medium does not provide the visual benefits that VC offers but is an inexpensive, ubiquitous, and reliable medium for communication. As with VC, telephone systems may make use of standard analog or digital voice connections (e.g., ISDN). Satellite or cellular communications may also be available for use in remote areas. Voice over Internet protocol (VoIP) may be attractive because of low cost, but as with much of the Internet, caution must be exercised because some VoIP lines fail to meet privacy and security requirements for health care. As mentioned earlier in this chapter, a serious problem with using telephones for service delivery is that many insurance carriers will not reimburse for telephone-based behavioral health care.

WEB-BASED APPLICATIONS (eHEALTH)

As part of TMH, other aspects of the Internet may also be used effectively for behavioral interventions. Although gaining traction in the United States (for more information visit the International Society for Research on Internet Interventions website, http://isrii.org/), eHealth treatment models have been shown to be effective in behavioral and mental health applications in many other countries worldwide (Andersson & Cuijpers, 2009; Cuijpers et al., 2009). Such eHealth approaches tend to be highly structured; self-guided or partly guided by the consumer/patient; personalized to the user; interactive; enhanced by graphics, animations, audio, and video; and tailored to provide follow-up and feedback (Ritterband et al., 2003). In general, coaching or therapist support (on-site, by VC, or over the telephone), paired with the online content, improves patient adherence and outcomes (Mohr, Burns, Schueller, Clarke, & Klinkman, 2013). Some eHealth approaches have managed to reduce psychotherapy staff time by 75% while delivering better outcomes than in-person care (Benton, Snowden, Heesacker, & Lee, 2015). Web-based programs may also be used for providing and administering remote psychological assessments and other behavioral measures. Internet-based testing and assessments can make use of enhancements such as multimedia content (i.e., pictures, videos, sounds), computer adaptive testing techniques, and automatic scoring and interpretation algorithms (see Luxton, Pruitt, & Osenbach, 2014).

MOBILE DEVICES

Mobile devices (i.e., smartphones and tablets) have capabilities for both synchronous and asynchronous telehealth. Smartphone and tablet devices that have video camera capabilities may be used as a mobile VC device (Luxton, McCann, Bush, Mishkind, & Reger, 2011) if electronic data security requirements are met. This increases the potential sites of service for both the client/patient and provider, and because mobile devices do not require fixed geographic locations, they provide opportunities for TMH care that is low cost, flexible, and mobile. However, wireless devices must generally use either cellular or Wi-Fi network connections, and thus video connection quality will depend on available bandwidth (Luxton, Mishkind, Crumpton, et al., 2012).

Smartphones can be used to provide communication between clients/patients via text messaging (Kim & Jeong, 2007; Kubota, Fujita, & Hatano, 2004) or with mobile health apps with communication features. The immediacy of these interventions in the real world offers new potential, including opportunities for near ubiquitous connection between a care system and a client/patient (Mohr et al., 2013). Text messages are often a piece of a larger behavioral or mental health intervention and include a range of information, such as psychoeducational messages, reminders, generic tips, and/or individualized feedback and encouragement.

Many smartphones have the capability to connect to external hardware devices such as biofeedback sensors for monitoring physiological signals. Newer aspects of such technology involve the *quantified self*, which is a movement supported by an ever-increasing array of smart device apps that allow the user to acquire a broad range of data pieces about the themselves (e.g., mood, sleep, activity, food intake) by self-tracking and auto-analytics, whereby the user is empowered by mobile technology to quantify his or her own biometrics and compare them to the biometrics of millions of other people (Lupton, 2013). Similarly, the rapid evolution of the Internet of Things, or IoT, allows users to interconnect mobile and computerized devices (e.g., sensors) that can communicate with each other via the Internet.

SELECTING APPROPRIATE TECHNOLOGIES FOR TELEMENTAL HEALTH

A checklist of steps to consider when selecting technologies includes the following:

- identify and match appropriate technology for the objective/task,
- determine whether the medium meets approved technical/privacy standards (see Chapter 3),
- assess whether feasible and acceptable for the TMH purpose (both from practitioner and client perspectives),
- consider the ability and need of the technology to support evidence-based protocols, and
- understand reimbursement relevant to the context and the technology.

First and foremost, the technology needs to fit the clinical objectives. For example, if it is important to see the client/patient, then VC will likely be the preferred option. In other applications, such as follow-up with patients, the telephone may be adequate for accomplishing clinical care goals, but reimbursement may be more difficult to obtain. Additionally, when working in high-demand situations with few trained clinicians, using evidence-based eHealth behavioral strategies to augment or replace direct care can increase access to care and associated relief of suffering for millions of persons who would otherwise not receive care or simply be placed on potentially problematic psychotropic medication without behavioral intervention by allied health professionals. Matching the technology to the clinical need, then, is primary.

Choosing an appropriate technology will also involve which technologies are available (e.g., at a hospital or group setting) and relevant local policies. Some organizations prohibit all e-mail or text messaging, for example. Ultimately, chosen technologies must meet both practitioner and patient preferences. That is, TMH practitioners should use technology for which they have all needed competencies to follow all relevant best ethical practices in assessment and treatment (see Chapter 3). Client/patient preferences must also be considered (American Psychological Association, 2013a), as well as equitable access to TMH services (Nelson, Davis, & Velasquez, 2012).

Selected technology must also meet technical standards, including electronic privacy requirements (see Chapter 3). *Bandwidth* refers to the rate (and thus amount) of information transmitted across the medium. In general, the amount of information to be transmitted in real time determines bandwidth requirements. VC, which involves both video data and voice data, will require more bandwidth than just a voice signal. The American Telemedicine Association's (2009) *Practice Guidelines for Videoconferencing-Based Telemental Health* recommends 384 Kbps or higher transmission speed to ensure "the smooth and natural communication pace necessary for clinical encounters" (p. 14). This minimum is a good rule of thumb but can vary with the types of software being used (video compression and other technologies). Some VC technologies also adjust bandwidth depending on quality of the connection. Although the connection is maintained, the quality may be diminished.

TMH practitioner technology choices must also match local population capacities. For example, a practitioner working in the North Dakota frontier may only have access to mobile telephone systems and e-mail. If using Apple's FaceTime video chat service, then, it would be his or her responsibility to learn and implement privacy and security protocols for this technology. Recommended activities include a thorough review of the American Telemedicine Association (2009) guidelines' technical specifications, as well as a review of a sponsoring organization's internal policies and procedures when choosing technology. As previously discussed, obtaining a written Business Associate's Agreement (BAA) is always required by HIPAA. A BAA is a contract between a HIPAA-covered entity (e.g., hospitals, clinics, health insurance providers) and a HIPAA business associate (any organization or person working in association with or providing services to a covered entity).

TMH practitioners should also use their judgment when deciding whether the bandwidth is adequate for providing clinical services. In situations where clinical judgment warrants a deviation from the previously described requirements, ample documentation for clinical justification is also strongly suggested. For instance, a clinical note may state,

> Jill's computer malfunctioned today. Given her distress with regard to the sudden death of her husband last week and ensuing family turmoil, she requested telephone sessions for therapy. No other technology was available to her at the time. As discussed during the informed consent process upon intake, she was offered the option of meeting with the therapist in person but declined the six-hour drive.

OPTIMIZING TELEHEALTH EQUIPMENT

With the wide range of technology currently available, clinicians need to be aware of best practices for optimizing equipment that they wish to use in their practice. Teleproviders should keep in mind that other VC issues present both strengths and weaknesses in seeing the client/patient, and these must be weighed from an ethical–legal perspective. On the one hand, the clinician must acknowledge that using VC eliminates full-body view of a client/patient. The loss of information from such limited view can influence how one works as a clinician, particularly if noting and commenting on body movement or lack thereof is an integral part of one's therapeutic focus. On the other hand, some VC equipment allows the clinician to zoom in unobtrusively and observe small movements such as possible tics that may not be visible in traditional settings. Tearing, tremors, and other small movements can also be detected with a zoom lens, but best practice dictates that patients are informed ahead of time when such equipment is to be used.

Further, using a mobile tablet or smartphone may make it difficult for the provider to see small client/patient details, facial expressions, and grooming. The TMH practitioner's monitor should be large enough to see sufficient detail necessary for the provider to make clinical decisions necessary for that particular encounter. Screen size may be especially important if conducting group therapy with VC when there are multiple people in the frame. Again, for some purposes a screen as large as a 52-inch television screen may be needed; in other cases, a tablet monitor is sufficient for the clinical or psychoeducational purpose. As long as the client/patient site has high definition camera equipment, the image resolution should support a clear picture on the clinician's monitor. Large monitors can also help reduce eyestrain and fatigue in clinicians who are practicing via technology for several hours in a row.

The placement of monitors in relation to seating and note taking equipment may also warrant consideration. Some telepractitioners choose to use standing desks, for example, to improve blood flow and alertness during long clinical hours. On the basis of telepractitioner preferences, video monitors can easily be arranged so that clients/patients will not notice and therefore be distracted by a clinician's choice to be standing or seated during sessions. When using mobile devices, clinicians may need to build or purchase a stand for mounting a smartphone to free a hand for note-taking.

TMH practitioners may also wish to view electronic health records concurrent with the clinical session. The use of multiple monitors may be helpful on the provider end, particularly when viewing the EHR or other information required during the VC session. As mentioned previously, a PIP configuration is another option that allows practitioners to see themselves in a small corner of their own video monitor. A PIP can be very helpful in allowing clinicians to view what patients are seeing, such as if they are off camera, poorly groomed, or have food in their teeth, or if something in their background looks unprofessional, such as crying children fighting in the hallway when the clinician's door is inadvertently left open in a home-based office. Note that using an additional monitor may prove less distracting for the provider.

Video cameras at both the patient and provider sites should be of sufficient resolution to capture detailed images. Any high-definition camera should provide acceptable resolution. Cameras with pan, tilt, and zoom capabilities may help to view the client/patient's location during clinical encounters if the client/patient is in a clinical setting. Additionally, the clinician will have little control of a camera's features when the client/patient is using his or her own equipment from a nonclinic setting, such as the home or office using laptops and integrated desktops with built-in cameras, such as Apple monitors. Also, lighting may need to be adjusted (e.g., moving a lamp, opening or closing window coverings) to ensure that the patient's face (and that of the teleprovider) is sufficiently illuminated.

Camera placement is another important consideration. Smaller screens with cameras located at the top of the screen may force the client/patient to gaze downward to see the clinician during interaction, thus making it more difficult to interpret facial expressions. Adaptive devices are available, such as mirrors that allow the clinician to look at the image of a patient on his or her own screen, but seemingly have eye contact when viewed from the patient screen. The field of telepresence is well documented and worth some focus by the conscientious teleprovider. Although minimum screen sizes do not seem to have been suggested by any large professional group, some employers and other organizations may specify minimum screen sizes. The patient site should also have a video monitor with an adequate size; smaller screens may force the patient to gaze downward, thus making it more difficult to interpret facial expressions.

Microphones and speakers should be of sufficient quality to assure effective communication. Microphone placement is important to consider so that speech is captured accurately. Microphones should be placed close enough to the person(s) speaking during the encounter to accurately capture voice sounds. Noise cancellation software is also quite helpful in noisy environments. When microphones fail, the clinician may consider muting sound that comes from the VC equipment and simply calling the client/patient on the telephone. Of the two signals, voice is the most important to capture accurately in most cases. Therapy can conceivably continue without video but must be stopped in the absence of an audio signal when conducted between individuals who cannot read lips. In the home-based setting, technical "test" connections are encouraged ahead of clinical encounters to evaluate audio and video quality and problem solve difficulties ahead of time. In some cases, specialized speaker/microphone devices can be tremendously helpful. For instance, Phoenix speakers can minimize ambient sound, maximize voice quality, and even allow hard-of-hearing patients to hold the device to their ear to facilitate nonintrusive communication.

Clinicians will do well to speak to their video conferencing service providers (video vendors) to determine the vendor's needs for optimal connectivity. Once they have assured themselves that their own equipment meets those specifications, they can share this information with their patients/clients. However, it is best to avoid bringing more stress on patients who may be distraught by burdening them with a list of technical specifications to decipher or making sure their equipment matches those needs. Oftentimes, experimenting with a patient who is willing to tinker with technology during an initial, unreimbursed session is the best route to reliable technical connections when using equipment as an independent practitioner. Agencies, clinics, and hospitals usually hire information technology professionals whose job it is to optimize connectivity.

BACKUP TECHNOLOGIES

Although most VC technologies are highly reliable, a backup plan should be included in the telepractice protocol (see Chapter 5) and shared with the client/patient at consent. Most commonly, a telephone provides an alternate means of communication should a loss of a VC connection occur. A phone can be used to contact technical support and also to reconnect patient and provider sites. Landline telephones may be most reliable; however, cellular or satellite telephones can also serve as adequate backups. In some settings, it may appropriate to use SMS texting or e-mail as a backup method for communication; however, use of these technologies should be based on local policies regarding their use and on personal preferences. Compliance with all local and federal security protocols must be in place for every device used. Checking with insurance companies reimbursing for such hybrid video/telephone sessions is also suggested.

3

Ethical, Legal, and Other Risk Management Considerations

The goal of most telemental health (TMH) services is to approximate the same best practices as in-office clinical care. In general, the same liabilities, risks, and ethical issues that are encountered during conventional in-office practice also apply to TMH (Kramer & Luxton, 2015; Kramer, Mishkind, Luxton, & Shore, 2013; Maheu, Pulier, Wilhelm, McMenamin, & Brown-Connolly, 2004). There are, however, several important and special considerations when engaging in TMH. These considerations generally center around two characteristics of TMH: geographical distance from the location of the client/patient and use of technology as the medium of service provision. These differences introduce additional risks and considerations that extend beyond those of conventional in-person services. This chapter provides the "need to know" information regarding legal, regulatory, ethical, liability, and related training issues in TMH practice.

http://dx.doi.org/10.1037/14938-004
A Practitioner's Guide to Telemental Health: How to Conduct Legal, Ethical, and Evidence-Based Telepractice, by D. D. Luxton, E.-L. Nelson, and M. M. Maheu

LICENSURE, SCOPE OF PRACTICE, AND LEGAL CONSIDERATIONS

Behavioral health care professionals engaged in telepractice must adhere to the requirements and restrictions of licensure, just as do those who practice in traditional in-person settings. This requires teleproviders to carefully consider their scope of practice specific to their license, as well as their individual training and experience. In addition, they must be cognizant of requirements when providing services across different jurisdictions.

In the United States, each state has control over establishing and enforcing licensure requirements of health care professionals, including behavioral health professionals (Health Resources and Services Administration, 2010). Every state has its own laws associated with the practice of health care within that state's boundaries, and laws are typically enforced by state regulatory boards. Certain federal government agencies (e.g., U.S. Department of Defense, Indian Health Services, Department of Veterans Affairs), however, allow some categories of health care providers licensed in one state to practice within their federal duties in any state (and sometimes across international borders), effectively allowing the licensure policy or regulation of the federal agency to preempt individual state licensure requirements (Kramer, Mishkind, Luxton, & Shore, 2013).

At the present time, and in most countries, legal and regulatory requirements are based on those in effect in the location of the client/patient at the time of the contact rather than those in effect in the location of the professional. It is therefore necessary for TMH professionals to be familiar with the applicable local (i.e., state or provincial) requirements of the originating site. In the United States, some states have specific telemedicine laws, and these laws vary from state to state in what type and under which circumstances care can be provided across state lines. Also, TMH services across state lines are potentially under the regulation of both the state where the provider is located and the state where the patient is located, so knowledge of more than just the state law of where the patient is located is essential. In some instances, it is also possible that a client/patient can bring a licensing complaint in either or both states (Barnett, Kelly, & Roberts, 2011; Kramer, Mishkind, Luxton, & Shore, 2013; Maheu et al., 2004). We recommend that providers exercise due diligence in exploring the current licensing laws in both their own and the client/patient's jurisdiction.

As of 2015, at least 26 U.S. states have some form of legislation regarding the practice of telehealth, and additional states have introduced or are considering telehealth legislation (American Psychological Association [APA], 2013b; see also http://cchpca.org/state-laws-and-reimbursement-policies). Many state telehealth laws address licensure requirements and their exceptions, such as the availability of temporary or limited licenses. Some require obtaining a full license to provide services within that state, whereas others offer consultations that allow an out-of-state licensed provider to consult with local providers serving patients in states where the consultant is unlicensed (Gupta & Sao, 2011). Some state laws apply to a broad range of telehealth services providers, and some specify a single type of provider (e.g., psychologist). Some discuss very specific requirements (e.g., informed consent) and some define which types of communication modalities are covered (e.g., telephone, e-mail, video). Moreover, some state statutes allow mental health professionals to practice within their state for a maximum number of days per year. They may provide some assurance for one who wishes to simply contact patients on a limited basis, when either the patient or provider is out of state because of work, education, or vacation. Compliance with all state and federal laws must be considered (see APA, 2010a).

In general, the safest risk management approach is to shoulder the financial and administrative burdens involved, but to obtain licenses in each state where one wishes to provide services. Programs established by groups to help ease such burdens are worthy of note, such as the Psychology Interjurisdictional Compact. The debate on potential licensing solutions continues (Kramer, Mishkind, Luxton, & Shore, 2013).

For up-to-date information regarding laws associated with TMH in the United States, readers may wish to visit the American Telemedicine Association's State Telemedicine Policy Center (available at http://www.americantelemed.org/) and its state telemedicine legislation tracking information. APA's (2013b) *Telepsychology 50-State Review* and the Federation of State Medical Board's (2013) *Telemedicine Overview: Board-by-Board Approach* are also valuable resources. Professionals in other countries may contact their professional associations or the consulate in the foreign nation to inquire about local authorities and how to contact for similar resources.

As in the on-site traditional setting, teleproviders carefully consider their scope of practice specific to their license, training, and experience. Such scope of practice is informed by statutes that are overseen by the state regulatory boards, as well as by professional organizations. Because telepractice may increase outreach to underserved populations with limited resources, it is not uncommon for TMH providers to become interested in expanding their practices. For example, a therapist who has mainly worked with adults may become interested in extending services to children and adolescents because no other services exist in the community. Teleproviders must give careful consideration to seeking the additional training and supervision necessary when expanding services to new populations or using new treatment approaches. Providers should also strive to be transparent concerning any conflict or perceived conflicts of interest when providing or recommending telepractice services if they own or have interests in related technology companies.

Some TMH practices may erroneously be promoted as "coaching" rather than licensed clinical interventions. The teleprovider should obtain and understand written descriptions of clinical and nonclinical services from their licensing board before making assumptions about legal definitions of regulated practice.

DUTY TO REPORT, DUTY TO WARN/PROTECT, AND CIVIL COMMITMENT

Familiarity with duty to report and duty to warn/protect (both statutory and case law requirements), as well as with civil commitment requirements, is also a necessity for TMH professionals. The requirements for duty to warn/protect as well as involuntary hospitalization vary by state

(Luxton, O'Brien, McCann, & Mishkind, 2012; Maheu et al., 2004). Moreover, some states do not have statutes or guidelines for duty to protect, and among the states that do have such statutes, there is substantial variability in language and expectations for behavioral health providers (Pabian, Welfel, & Beebe, 2009). Behavioral health professionals who are considering TMH should be aware of civil commitment and duty to warn/protect requirements in their jurisdiction as well as that of the client/patient (Shore, Bloom, Manson, & Whitener, 2008). Telemental health professionals should also be aware of applicable institutional level guidance and requirements that may address these issues. As in the in-office setting, teleproviders have responsibilities as mandated reporters and must be aware of their jurisdiction's requirements regarding vulnerable populations (e.g., children, elders). They should also be aware of legal and ethical considerations associated with disclosure of behaviors (e.g., sexual activity, substance use/abuse) to parents and guardians of adolescent patients, and families should be reminded of these requirements during the informed consent process. It is also important to engage the family to inform them of the process of mandated reporting and what to expect in terms of local follow-up. As in the on-site setting, the teleprovider assesses any imminent threat of harm to the child as a result of the disclosure and engages law enforcement assistance if needed. In supervised TMH settings, site coordinators should follow preestablished protocols to support the teleprovider as he or she advises the family of the reportable concern and joins with the family around a treatment plan. In the home-based TMH setting, careful consideration should be given to risks associated with disclosure of these behaviors (e.g., a patient who may become violent toward family members).

PRIVACY AND DATA SECURITY CONSIDERATIONS

Ensuring that patient privacy and data security are compliant with federal and state or provincial laws needs to be a priority for TMH professionals. These laws often require more than the purchase of equipment that meets standards set by the authorities; they can also involve a set of processes that one must use (Maheu et al., 2004). For instance, in the United States, the Health Insurance Portability and Accountability Act of 1996 (HIPAA) requires that clinicians educate their staff, conduct regular risk assessments for all technologies used, have written breach remediation plans, and more (visit the U.S. Department of Health and Human Services website for more information about these HIPAA requirements http://www.hhs.gov/ocr/privacy/; also http://www.apapracticecentral.org/business/hipaa/breach-notification.aspx). Site coordinators assisting at the client/patient site, especially those who are new to behavioral and mental health encounters, should be trained to the expected levels of privacy and security. For example, an untrained coordinator in a small rural community could violate these expectations by looking at a file of a neighbor or asking a fellow parishioner about an upcoming clinical appointment. Clinicians and their employers will also want to consult with an attorney familiar with telehealth to make sure that all involved state laws are being followed, because state law can build on and surpass federal laws with additional requirements.

Awareness of these laws is important given the diversity and rapid evolution of technologies (e.g., videoconferencing [VC], Internet, mobile apps) available for TMH. For example, using smart devices or websites to collect client/patient assessment data requires different security features than required for VC alone. Some Internet or mobile device applications may not meet minimum requirements for data security, and data may be collected by or stored by third parties, thus posing privacy risks (Luxton, Kayl, & Mishkind, 2012). Staying current with all these laws is also important. For instance, the HIPAA Omnibus rule enacted in 2013 has increased requirements as well as fines and other consequences for HIPAA noncompliance (Kramer & Luxton, 2015). Providers and their employers using technology must make wise choices with technology because they now are partially responsible if the technology causes damages to clients/patients. Although Business Associate Agreements (BAAs) are now required, they do not absolve the clinician or employer of all responsibility in the event consumers are harmed. HIPAA requires that a number of standards be met, including the availability of "audit trails" that make records of interactions accessible to authorities when needed. HIPAA also requires "breach notification tools" to inform clinicians of breaches, such as when a transmission is illegally hacked. There continues to be debate on whether the use of commercially available products, such as Skype, are HIPAA compliant (Maheu & McMenamin, 2013), but large American mental health membership associations such as the National Association of Social Workers (2008) and APA (2013a) have issued statements warning their members of the dangers of using such technologies. Also, many professionals also do not realize that federal laws (i.e., HIPAA in the United States; the Personal Information Protection and Electronic Documents Act in Canada) only establish a "floor" for minimum privacy and security requirements when transmitting data. States and provinces can add significant additional requirements for professionals.

Moreover, institutions may have concerns related to such products separate from HIPAA, such as network security risks associated with VC that uses third-party servers. Some VC software applications may use network servers to run the VC software, and if these servers are hosted and controlled by a third party, there may be concern by institutions as to whether the required level of security is being met (e.g., physical security of the servers, firewall protection to protect from hackers).

The first step in risk management associated with privacy and data security is learn the appropriate rules (for a resource, see the American Medical Association's summary of the new HIPAA rules: http://www.ama-assn.org/resources/doc/washington/hipaa-omnibus-final-rule-summary.pdf). This assessment is important because providers may be working with outside institutions with different electronic health record systems or, in some rural/remote areas, continuing to use paper charts. Clinicians must be explicit concerning where the designated medical record resides and who has access to the record at the clinician site and at the presenting site (e.g., rural hospital, clinic, school). Formal risk assessment is also required by the 2013 HIPAA Omnibus Act. These assessments can be easily conducted and at no cost by using the U.S. Department of Health & Human Services' Security Risk Assessment Tool (see http://www.healthit.gov/providers-professionals/security-risk-assessment). In addition, there are a several guidelines and other TMH resources specific to HIPAA compliance, appropriate technology to use, and methods to safeguard data security and patient privacy (Kramer, Mishkind, Luxton, & Shore, 2013; Luxton, Kayl, & Mishkind, 2012; Turvey et al., 2013). Legal consultation is recommended whenever there is uncertainty about privacy and data security requirements.

In addition to technology-related security, the teleprovider should consider room-related privacy in both the provider and the distant settings and strive to provide the same in-office standards for professionalism. This includes ensuring that individuals cannot easily see or hear into the teleconferencing room. There is less direct provider control over the client/patient's environment. The provider may want to ask the client/patient and site coordinator if anyone else is in the room, as well as to scan the room remotely using the telemedicine camera when these capabilities are available and with the knowledge and consent of the patient. The site coordinator may assist with managing the flow of individuals in and out of the room to decrease the potential for eavesdropping at the door, for example, directing a teen to the waiting room as the parent talks independently with the therapist or vice versa. In unsupervised settings, the teleprovider should talk with the client/patient about where in the home or other environment is most private. If there are many people coming and going from the room or other unexpected interruptions, a different room should be used.

INFORMED CONSENT REQUIREMENTS

Informed consent is the process whereby the recipient of care is given adequate information to make an informed choice about the care to be received. This process is generally considered a necessary and ethical standard of care when initiating any behavioral health treatment. It often is both a legal requirement and an ethical mandate. It therefore is recommended that TMH professionals in every discipline review applicable informed consent regulations in all relevant states and countries for a specific list of required consent elements. Furthermore, professional associations may need to be consulted to fully understand discipline-specific standards of care related to informed consent.

Employers may also add requirements. For instance, large federal government organizations such as the U.S. Department of Veterans Affairs and the U.S. military health care system have created sample informed consent forms for telehealth, and many additional templates are available through the Telehealth Resource Centers, the American Telemedicine Association, and other organizations. Although sample informed consent documents are available online, they always need final review by an attorney who is knowledgeable of local relevant laws. Specific populations to be addressed by telehealth service may also need to be reflected in these documents. When preceded by adequate preparation by the clinician, such legal consultations can be quite cost-effective.

Guidelines from professional associations should also be consulted to fully understand specific discipline-specific standards of care related to informed consent. For example, Guideline 3 of APA's (2013a) *Guidelines for the Practice of Telepsychology* states

> Psychologists strive to obtain and document informed consent that specifically addresses the unique concerns related to the telepsychology services they provide. When doing so, psychologists are cognizant of the applicable laws and regulations, as well as organizational requirements that govern informed consent in this area.

Guideline 3 (APA, 2013a) also states

> When developing such informed consent, psychologists make reasonable effort to use language that is reasonably understandable to their clients/patients, in addition to, evaluating the need to address cultural, linguistic, organizational considerations, and other issues that may impact on a client/patient's understanding of the informed consent agreement. When considering for inclusion in informed consent those unique concerns that may be involved in providing telepsychology services, psychologists may include the manner in which they and their clients/patients will use the particular telecommunication technologies, the boundaries they will establish and observe, and the procedures for responding to electronic communications from clients/patients.

As in any informed consent process, the teleprovider gains a clear understanding of the relationships with those participating in the consent process, including legal guardianship and legal capacity of the individual to consent to treatment. In addition to informed consent procedures, teleproviders often ask clients/patients to complete their organization's HIPAA-related Notice of Privacy Plan.

The American Telemedicine Association's guidelines (Turvey et al., 2013) have also highlighted the importance of obtaining informed consent with patients in real time. Those guidelines provide some recommended elements for informed consent (in the absence of specific law or regulation), that include the following:

- confidentiality and limits to confidentiality when using electronic communications;
- emergency plan and contact information for local resources;
- process for documentation and storage of information;
- potential for technical failure and procedures for coordination of care with other professionals; protocol for contact between sessions; and
- conditions under which TMH services are terminated and a referral for face-to-face care made.

All of the standard components of informed consent used in traditional care should be included. There are a few additional specifics that should be communicated. It is important to describe the technology to be used and what its use entails. This description should also include the risks and benefits of using the technology for remote services. It is also a good practice to articulate expectations for scheduling, frequency of communication, as well as use of other communication methods (e.g., policies on texting or e-mailing). We discuss these recommendations in more detail in the following paragraphs.

RISKS AND EXPECTATIONS

The TMH informed consent should include additional elements that describe risks associated with technology, privacy, and managing emergencies. Ideally, the informed consent is a springboard to a welcoming conversation between the client/patient and provider to address questions and concerns that the client/patient may have both about the technology and about the behavioral health process in general. At the beginning of the encounter, it is a good idea to talk with clients/patients about their path to the telepractice clinic, to make sure that they are aware of both on-site and telepractice options and that they are choosing to be seen over technology. It is also important to describe the technology to be used in easy-to-understand language, what its use entails, and what expectations are regarding its use. Children should be reassured that the VC is like a phone call with a picture and not like watching TV, emphasizing "only the therapist can see you and only you can see the therapist; no one else can see us talking."

The informed consent should include a description of expectations for scheduling, frequency of communication, attendance policies, and use of other communication methods (such as policy on texting or e-mailing). Regardless of whether the clinician is comfortable with using e-mail or texting for professional practice, the patient may attempt to use these media to establish contact with the clinician. Thus, it is essential for the clinician to include related policies during the informed consent process. If a trainee is involved with the delivery of services, information about the trainee and the trainee's supervision should be shared in the informed consent process. If there are any financial considerations unique to telepractice, such as room fees required by the distant site, these are disclosed. It is necessary to inform clients/patients of the limits to confidentiality and risks to the possible access or disclosure of confidential data and information that may occur during service delivery, including the risks of access to electronic communications (e.g., telephone, e-mail) between the telepractitioner and client/patient (APA, 2013a). The provider should also provide rationales for limiting e-mail interaction, including concerns about how to verify the identity of the sender and limitations to the speed of response.

The informed consent process also advises the client/patient of other security precautions taken by the clinician, such as adherence to all state and federal laws, the clinician's policies regarding notifying the client/patient if breaches occur, the use of passwords on all computers and devices, and procedures for downloading of text messages and e-mail to the client/patient's record.

Disclosure should be made as to how electronic data are stored and disposed of, as well as whether the sessions are to be recorded. Moreover, a separate written approval and consent is essential if the telepractitioner intends to videotape a session, including information concerning whether this recording will become part of the medical record. The reader is also encouraged to include a social media policy statement, which may be brief and all inclusive. If "friending" clients/patients is not within the scope of services provided, a clear statement can be included in the informed consent discussion to reflect such boundaries.

It is also important to consider technical feasibility, as technical issues may increase liability. If the clinician knows that technical difficulties are probable (e.g., given network connectivity problems or user inexperience with technology), it may be wise to seek an alternative.

EMERGENCIES

Full disclosure of policies and procedures for clinical emergencies is necessary, as is informing patients that they have an option to refuse TMH care and, if they do refuse, that they retain the option of receiving face-to-face care (Kramer, Mishkind, Luxton, & Shore, 2013). A description of the roles of each party (e.g., provider, client/patient, caregivers, and/or staff at remote site) during care and emergency management should be provided, as well as ongoing training to ensure staff are aware and can provide the emergency support. Emergency plans may also include descriptions of when remote emergency resources will be accessed. For example, "A client/patient's emergency contact person (e.g., family member, friend, and/or physician) will be contacted immediately if there is reason to believe that there is imminent danger to the client/patient or any other individual(s) in their environment." Written protocols may also include descriptions of security measures to assure compliance with relevant federal and state laws related to the release and sharing of information (e.g., consent forms, assessment materials) between locations. For more details on what to include in an emergency plan, see Chapter 5 of this volume.

It is important to periodically review the emergency procedures, particularly because of the high turnover of staff and instability in resources in some underserved settings. Also, as specifically stated in the *Guidelines for the Practice of Telepsychology* (APA, 2013a),

> psychologists may need to be aware of the manner in which cultural, linguistic, socioeconomic characteristics, and organizational considerations may impact a client/patient's understanding of, and the special considerations required for, obtaining informed consent (such as when securing informed consent remotely from a parent/guardian when providing telepsychology services to a minor).

The legal rights of the child and adolescent are paramount and may vary depending on circumstance (e.g., age, foster status). It is best practice to confirm that whoever has legal right to be included in treatment, with or without the child's consent in an in-person environment, is also afforded the same right during TMH services.

LIMITATIONS

TMH practitioners need to inform clients/patients about the potential limitations or risks of providing behavioral and mental health services with telehealth technologies. Limitations to crisis intervention should also be disclosed. It may be prudent to disclose the following limitations and risks:

- an emerging scientific telepractice literature that has some limitations;
- a lack of nonverbal cues (when using voice-only technologies);
- e-mail and SMS messages may not be received or may be delayed;
- the professional may not be available to respond within the desired time frame or may designate another provider to respond during the primary provider's absence (e.g., vacation, medical or family leave);
- the need for a particular level of technical specification (e.g., computer or network infrastructure);

- information may be forwarded inadvertently to a wrong address or number; and
- other people may access clients'/patients' e-mail, of which the clinician has no control.

Further, because TMH services may require the identification of a support person at the distant site, disclosure of risks to privacy when engaging with third parties should be disclosed and discussed as part of the informed consent process. Moreover, requirements for duty to warn should also be provided.

Last, it is crucial to note that informed consent can differ from one state or country to another. Astute practitioners take nothing for granted, allocating the hour or two necessary to research each foreign state or country's website to look for listings of required informed consent elements and contacting regulatory boards for information about informed consent requirements when applicable. Professional training in the form of courses, webinars, or in-person trainings are currently available both online and in person to address informed consent. Additionally, consultation with appropriately trained legal counsel is recommended. Membership associations may also be organized to help recruit such specialty consultation at reasonable costs for small group and independent practitioners.

MALPRACTICE INSURANCE: DO YOU NEED IT TO PROVIDE TELEMENTAL HEALTH?

Many states require a health care professional to have malpractice insurance if providing care in their state. In addition, many malpractice insurance companies have established policies that were designed to cover traditional in-office encounters within the state where the professional practices and is licensed. For federal government employees, that requirement is usually met through coverage under the Federal Tort Claims Act (28 U.S.C. 1346(b)), which protects government employees from personal liability by substituting the U.S. government as a defendant in any case brought against them for care provided in their federal employment.

TMH professionals should verify that their insurance covers telemedicine services and that their professional liability insurance covers them in all the states in which they practice and intend to provide services. When considering an insurance plan, a thorough review of the coverage is recommended to determine the inclusion of coverage for telemedicine or any mention of coverage for care provided in another state. It may be necessary to contact malpractice insurance carriers to clarify any concerns or unknowns, obtain their clarifications in writing, and perhaps bring them to an attorney to make sure all benefits are enforceable. Problems can arise. Some companies have been known to offer telehealth coverage for inexpensive regulatory suits but not potentially more expensive civil suits or fail to clearly inform policyholders when their coverage can be nullified, such as when practicing in a state that considers some infractions to be "criminal" in intent.

WHEN YOU HAVE QUESTIONS ABOUT LIABILITIES AND RISKS

State or provincial professional boards are a potential resource for clarifying what regulations may or may not apply when providing care in a particular jurisdiction. Some have issued written opinions addressing what services require a license. Telehealth-savvy attorneys are suggested, rather than the typical business attorney often available through one's professional association to navigate subpoenas or rental leases. Legal counsel who is familiar with telehealth issues can assist in helping to fully research the issues and offer legal opinions based on his or her research and knowledge (Maheu et al., 2004). For example, if the teleprovider is prescribing scheduled medications, he or she is encouraged to consult legal counsel about the most recent local, state, and federal laws that may require seeing a client/patient first in person. It is also strongly suggested that practitioners and their employers check with a distant state or country professional boards before providing service in foreign locations. Ample time may need to be allotted for written communication to confirm whether local laws need to be followed and to obtain any written policies regarding local definitions of legal practice within that state or country. Related resources are available through the Telehealth Resource Centers (http://www.telehealthresourcecenter.org/).

When initiating telepractice, providers are encouraged to obtain professional education, supervision, and/or consultation as per ethical requirements. Mentorship in the clinical, technical, and outreach/community engagement components associated with telehealth may also be beneficial (Nelson, Bui, & Sharp, 2011). As in on-site services, professional training, ongoing supervision, and peer-to-peer support are important components in providing high-quality care and in risk management (APA, 2010a). When possible, it can be very helpful to shadow an established TMH provider before beginning practice and considering approaches to these ethical/legal components, including risk management. Often in traditional telehealth models with established sites (e.g., large teaching hospitals), supervision systems may be in place, in-house staff may assist with technical challenges, and emergency backup protocols may be well established. However, consideration should be given to ongoing training as new personnel come onboard, to updating protocols on the basis of technology updates and input from multiple informants (e.g., clinicians, presenters, patients), and to tailoring protocols when working with diverse distant sites.

Behavioral health professionals who work in small and/or independent practices, however, may not enjoy the benefits of the aforementioned processes, resources, and professional support communities. To manage risk associated with providing TMH services in small clinics, group practices, or independently, careful preparation and professional training will decrease the burden experienced by individual practitioners. Such thoughtful preparation and support can also relieve the clinician's anxiety, inspire creative approaches to old problems, and improve the quality of the clinician's experience of practicing telehealth. Professional training is available in traditional in-person workshop formats as well as online through eLearning websites offering TMH training for continuing education hours.

4

Establishing a Telemental Health Practice

Because of their excitement over new technologies and their enthusiasm for extending services, providers are often eager to jump right to providing services. However, experience has shown that the most successful telepractices have taken the time to carefully identify and define program needs before beginning. A structured development process allows the provider to consider decisions and impact before making costly decisions (additional resources at http://www.hrsa.gov/publichealth/guidelines/behavioralhealth/behavioralhealthcareaccess.pdf). This chapter provides an overview of business planning and suggests additional resources for completing this in-depth process. The topics presented next are relevant for providers who either are interested in solely offering telemental health (TMH) services or who wish to augment their existing in-office services. This chapter informs providers working within a health care system as well as those who work alone or in group practices.

http://dx.doi.org/10.1037/14938-005
A Practitioner's Guide to Telemental Health: How to Conduct Legal, Ethical, and Evidence-Based Telepractice, by D. D. Luxton, E.-L. Nelson, and M. M. Maheu

NEEDS ASSESSMENT

Needs assessment supports the telepractitioner in identifying and assessing unmet clinical need in areas where he or she is considering practice and assessing individual and organizational readiness to meet these needs with telehealth. It includes data gathering about the prevalence of the behavioral condition within the target population as well as the service availability, often identified from federal (e.g., Health Resources Service Administration, Substance Abuse and Mental Health Services Administration, Centers for Disease Control's National Center for Health Statistics, Medicaid and Medicare reports) and regional (e.g., state and local health departments, community health assessments, community members, Telehealth Resource Centers) and other sources. If the provider is expanding services from an existing on-site practice, long wait times and patients/families driving miles for the particular behavioral treatment inform TMH focus. With existing practices, it is helpful to look at on-site referral patterns in identifying TMH partners.

The needs assessment also supports important relationship building with the local community. Ideally, it includes on-site conversations or focus groups with various stakeholders, including consumers and advocacy groups, local mental health professionals across settings and disciplines, primary care providers, and other formal and informal leaders (e.g., hospital administration or other community leaders). When feasible, it is a good idea to speak with payers about their interest in the new telepractice services. Other groups are relevant depending on the populations (e.g., schools, nursing facilities, substance abuse treatment). When on-site interactions are not feasible, telephone and video interactions are a good start. This process helps the provider identify where the demand for the service regularly exceeds local resources.

Remember that the goal of these early interactions is to listen and learn, reflecting genuine interest in how the provider can collaborate with the community to address a high need to use technology. As the provider builds relationships with the stakeholders, there is more detailed discussion of the proposed TMH service. These early conversations lay the foundation for the community engagement often needed to support the telepractitioner at a distance and gain buy-in from formal and informal community leaders. As the telepractice clinic "goes live," these supporters are invaluable in "getting the word out" to the community and helping develop a sustainable clinic.

Needs assessments include many stakeholder questions, focused on gathering data to answer "who, what, where, when, why, how" questions. The core components of needs assessment can form the beginning of a TMH business plan and are summarized as follows:

- *Why* are you providing the telepractice services?
  - What are the service gaps in a geographic area?
  - Who is the current and potential competition?
  - Which types of services will be most advantageous now? How does that differ from the types of services to be delivered 5 or 10 years from now?
  - Does the proposed service align with the organization's current vision, mission, and strategic plan?
  - Does the proposed service have a champion? Do stakeholders support the program? Can the leaders of key organizations be recruited to support the plan prior to its initiation?
- *Which* telepractice services best fit the need?
  - Which assessment services will be offered over videoconferencing?
  - Which treatment services will be provided?
  - Which consultation services will be provided?
  - Which telesupervision services will be provided?
- *Whom* will you serve?
  - Which populations, including age groups, will be served?
  - What specific behavioral presentations will be included and excluded?
- *Where* will the telepractice services be delivered?
  - How will TMH services be integrated with other care services (e.g., primary care, hospital, federally qualified health centers, certified community mental health clinics, and other settings)?
  - What equipment, infrastructure, and space are required and available for TMH services, both at the provider site(s) and the client/patient site(s)?

- *When* will the clinic be established and telepractice services initiated?
  - How much time will it take to find and set up the equipment and connectivity?
  - How much time is needed to develop TMH clinical skills?
  - How much time will be allocated for service delivery once initiated?
  - What are the plans for "scaling" the service? How will the often-logarithmic increase in service demand be met over time? How will services be documented?
  - How will the new service be promoted initially and over time?
  - How many clients can be expected in the first year, 2 years, 3 years, etc.?
- *How* will the new telepractice service be delivered?
  - How will new referral sources be cultivated now and in the future, as well as maintained over time?
  - How can potential opposition to the telepractice services be minimized?
  - How can competitors be minimized?

The needs assessment includes gathering information about existing resources and how they may support telepractice, as well as considerations of new resources. Readers are referred to other chapters as they have additional questions based on their unique situation. This encompasses; technical needs (Chapter 2); administrative and professional needs (Chapter 3), including licensing, credentialing, and malpractice insurance; and emergency management needs (Chapter 5). There are also many resources to help telepractitioners learn about and complete telehealth needs assessment, such as the U.S. Department of Health and Human Services (http://www.hrsa.gov/healthit/toolbox/RuralHealthITtoolbox/Telehealth/howdoyoubegin.html), the Department of Defense (http://t2health.dcoe.mil/sites/default/files/TMH-Guidebook-Dec2013.pdf), and the federally funded Telehealth Resource Centers (http://www.telehealthresourcecenter.org/sites/main/files/file-attachments/complete-program-developer-kit-2014-web1.pdf), among others. For providers reaching out to underserved communities, the Community Toolbox provides additional insight (http://ctb.ku.edu/en).

BUSINESS PLANNING

Business planning goes hand-in-hand with needs assessment. It is essential for developing a plan for short- and long-term telepractice success. The needs assessment informs the resources that are needed across technologies, space, personnel, training, and marketing. A clear understanding of the proposed telepractice's financial impact is crucial, along with consideration of the risks associated with the implementation and decisions of the business model (Maheu, Whitten, & Allen, 2001; California Telehealth Resource Center, 2014). Careful attention should be given to whether one's organization is willing to implement telepractice if there is not a revenue positive or neutral program design, such as in the case of mission-driven services. The business plan includes estimates for service delivery, costs to develop and operate the behavioral service, and the sources of revenue. Costs for telehealth can be viewed from the perspective of the patients, the providers, and the client/patient site. Both start-up and operating costs should be taken into consideration, including who will pay for each component over time.

The following are important economic aspects to consider when establishing a practice (see Luxton, 2013):

- potential cost reductions (e.g., providers no longer traveling to remote clinics);
- costs for equipment, software, upgrades, office space, and network infrastructure;
- use of personally owned devices (patient's computer/webcams, etc.) versus need to purchase equipment;
- personnel costs across technical support, scheduling, billing, and general administrative supports;
- costs for specialized clinical training and documentation to meet legal and ethical requirements; general costs associated with the clinic including promotional/marketing materials, paperwork, behavioral questionnaires and scoring, clinic-specific materials (e.g., a scale may be of interest in a health psychology clinic), electronic health records, etc.;
- attorney and accounting fees;

- costs associated with distant site support of the patient, including a telemedicine coordinator when applicable;
- expected client/patient volume and payer mix, including planning for often-seen patterns of logarithmic growth as the telepractice is established;
- consideration of funding sources across insurers, contractual arrangements with sites, grants, philanthropy, institutional investment, and other potential sources;
- costs associated with internal quality improvement or other evaluation; and
- external economic factors such as inflation, interest rates, depreciation, changes in technology costs, etc.

A plan to track data to determine costs over time is recommended. Some large institutions and health care systems may already have a process for cost capture in place; however, the independent practitioner or group practices will need to establish a process for cost capture. More formal economic evaluation techniques can be used to determine the number of sessions to offset technology and staffing costs (see Luxton, 2013; see also Chapter 6, this volume).

REIMBURSEMENT

Before delivering service, the telepractitioner may benefit from knowing the details of reimbursement. In the United States and at the time of this writing, federal government insurance reimbursement for Medicare is available for many disabled retired Americans.[1] The Medicare program is under the purview of the Centers for Medicare and Medicaid Services (CMS). These programs will reimburse only for telehealth services delivered under strict guidelines. The patients must be presented from an originating site situated in a rural Health Professional Shortage Area (HPSA), located either outside of a Metropolitan Statistical Area (MSA)

[1] The authors have gone into some detail about the CMS programs because in the United Sates, many other insurance programs follow precedents set by CMS. Other countries have different payment systems so the delineation may be irrelevant.

or in a rural census tract, or in a county outside of an MSA. A federal website tool (https://www.cms.gov/telehealth/) assists in determining eligibility as a potential originating sites. In addition, the Telehealth Resource Centers (http://www.telehealthresourcecenter.org/reimbursement) are available for technical assistance. Several other conditions must be met for Medicare payments to be made for telehealth services. Specifically, the service must be on the list of covered Medicare telehealth services and meet all of the following requirements for coverage: The service must be delivered via an interactive telecommunications system to someone eligible for Medicare services; the practitioner furnishing the service must meet the telehealth requirements, as well as the usual Medicare requirements; and the individual receiving the services must be located at an eligible originating site. When all of these conditions are met, Medicare reimburses an "originating site" fee to the originating site and provides separate payment to the distant-site practitioner delivering the service. State Medicaid policies often follow Medicare guidance, but there is variability in specific requirements from state to state. Private insurers also tend to follow CMS regarding coverage but may have additional requirements for telehealth coverage.

For TMH assessment-related reimbursement through CMS, the telehealth service must generally be delivered via an interactive telecommunications system. Under the definition of *telehealth services* given by CMS (§410.78(a)(3), 2011), an *interactive telecommunications system* is defined as multimedia communications equipment that includes, . . . *at a minimum, audio and video equipment permitting two-way, real-time interactive communication between the patient and distant site physician or practitioner* (MS-1612-FC 187) (Telehealth Services, 2011). VC communication equipment must also meet all legal requirements for privacy and security.

Initial intake and associated assessment over VC is often reimbursed, within the reimbursement constraints addressed in other chapters. Nonetheless, many types of clinical assessments are conducted as part of typical TMH clinical care services in varied settings and situations. For example, the measurement of clinical symptoms for the assessment of treatment progress is quite common during TMH clinical treatment services (Luxton, Pruitt, & Osenbach, 2014).

PROTOCOLS

The needs assessment and business plan provide the road map for developing detailed protocols and procedures for the telepractice clinic. Protocols are practical documents describing the processes and each individual's role before, during, and after a telepractice consultation—in particular, how the telepractice clinic can ensure that proper procedures for documentation, staffing credentials and competencies, and patient privacy are followed. Protocols also include a plan for coordinating with staff at the remote site, troubleshooting technical problems, and managing clinical/medical emergencies (see Chapter 5 for more information). Alternate contact methods, such as by telephone, are necessary to maintain a connection between the patient and originating site and to contact technical support. In addition, protocols outline how electronic data and information remain accessible in the event of technical difficulties.

Protocols detail the telepractice workflow, including similarities and differences from the on-site setting. They help make sure best practices are implemented in the telehealth setting, and telepractices may consider protocol checklists to assist in understanding what is working as well as areas of improvement within the new clinic. In general, telepractice policies and procedures should approximate the in-office setting. Consideration should be given to the additional administrative demands required in some TMH practice models, including the scheduling demands when coordinating across numerous TMH providers and many sites, as well as billing staff well-versed in telehealth requirements. A process for ongoing provider, presenter, technical and administrative staff, and patient feedback should be established to continuously improve the protocol and match to evolving needs.

TELEPRACTICE CHAMPIONS AND DISTANT SITE COORDINATORS/PRESENTERS

For telepractices that are delivering services in supervised settings (e.g., hospitals, clinics, schools, prisons), it is important to identify a telepractice "champion" at the distant site. Ideally, the champion is a trusted leader within the organization and someone with telehealth experiences. This "point person's" enthusiastic support lends credibility at the local level and can often be persuasive in convincing other local providers and agencies of the value of a new TMH clinic. The champion helps to gain buy-in both from the organization's leadership and administration and from clinic personnel who may be asked to expand their duties in support of the telepractice clinic.

In addition, a TMH site coordinator/TMH presenter/telefacilitator (American Telemedicine Association Telepresenting Standards and Guidelines Working Group, 2011; http://www.americantelemed.org/resources/nomenclature) is another crucial team member at the distant site. The role is often important in completing reimbursement requirements, such as verifying patient identity, confirming insurance coverage, collecting payment, and so forth. Sometimes the site champion and site coordinator are the same person. The site coordinator completes training to become proficient in both technology and behavioral health supports to meet the clinic needs. Qualifications for a telemedicine presenter include training as a health care professional (not necessarily behavioral health), technical proficiency and good communication skills, and a manner to make the patient and family comfortable throughout the telepractice session.

Site coordinators and other staff at the distant site (when available) may be responsible for a variety of helpful administrative, technical, and clinical tasks. The telepractitioner is encouraged to build strong relationships with these facilitators to jointly support the patient/family and to work together to resolve difficulties. As members of the client/patient's community, they can inform the provider of community-wide events that may impact the client/patient. The site coordinators assist as the extended "eyes and ears" of the telepractitioner and support all elements of the protocol before the session (with scheduling, paperwork, and socialization to the behavioral health system), during the session (with technical and clinical support, including assistance in emergency situations), and after the session (with understanding and implementing recommendations, including referrals). They orient patients/families to the telepractice and behavioral health processes, help complete the informed consent process, allay worries about the technology, and answer questions that the patient may have. With the patient's knowledge and consent, the telepractitioner guides the site coordinator in terms of when he or she is needed in the room.

Again, with consent, the site coordinator may also provide information on the patient's functioning across systems/situations. For example, when the site coordinator is a school nurse, he or she may be able to comment on the progress of strategies within the school setting. The coordinator may also administer screening measures and assess for signs that suggest TMH may not be appropriate for the client/patient and communicate those concerns to the provider (see Chapter 7). They may coordinate electronic retrieval and transfer of necessary records or documentation to the provider delivering the service prior to the visit. They may also be able to prepare the VC equipment and test it to make sure that it is working properly, as well as check that the room is prepared for clinical encounters. Another advantage of these staff is that they may remain on call during the clinical sessions to assist in case any clinical or medical emergency protocols are initiated (see Chapter 5). Further, they can handle other necessary end-of-visit documentation that may include arranging follow-up scheduling, completing satisfaction surveys, answering questions about referrals or other recommendations, or serving any other immediate needs the patient may have at the completion of the encounter to help ensure coordination and continuation of care.

PILOT TMH PROGRAMS

As a standard recommended when initiating new clinics, we encourage a continuous quality improvement approach (see Institute for Healthcare Improvement, http://www.ihi.org) when starting a telepractice. A pilot of the telepractice service can test the waters before full adoption (Shore & Manson, 2005). A pilot may involve a limited number of TMH visits for a specified period of time to evaluate what worked and what did not to inform decisions regarding expansion of TMH services. A pilot can be useful for testing technical procedures and troubleshooting as well as refining the scheduling and referral processes. Protocols and processes can be refined based on feedback.

5

Safety Planning and Emergency Management

This chapter provides an overview of safety issues encountered during telemental health (TMH) practice as well as the essential components required for safety plans and emergency protocols for TMH services. Safety planning is a necessary component of competent and ethical telepractice and a must for all practitioners across telepractice settings. Safety planning involves identifying steps and procedures for addressing situations that present a risk to the safety of clients/patients and other persons such as family members or clinical staff members during the course of telehealth services (Knapp, Younggren, VandeCreek, Harris, & Martin, 2013; Luxton, O'Brien, McCann, & Mishkind, 2012). In writing this chapter, we drew from the latest published standards and guidelines from professional organizations (e.g., American Counseling Association [ACA], American Association for Marriage and Family Therapy [AAMFT], American Psychological

http://dx.doi.org/10.1037/14938-006
A Practitioner's Guide to Telemental Health: How to Conduct Legal, Ethical, and Evidence-Based Telepractice, by D. D. Luxton, E.-L. Nelson, and M. M. Maheu

Association [APA], American Telemedicine Association [ATA]) and from the existing telehealth literature.

When conducted in accordance with evidence-based protocols (Luxton, Sirotin, & Mishkind, 2010), there is not any evidence that TMH, including home-based TMH, is less safe than traditional in-office services. However, the TMH practitioner's inquiries and interventions may be notably limited. Clinicians may do well to carefully consider the viability of specific techniques to both prevent and handle safety issues when working with distant populations. In some situations, TMH may offer additional safety because of the connections it affords across systems of care, allowing the consenting patient, behavioral health provider, and local health care professionals to work together around safety concerns.

The components of effective safety planning can be classified into the following general categories:

- assessment of the appropriateness for TMH services for the client/patient;
- assessment of client/patient's site factors;
- plan for coordinating with support persons and emergency services at originating sites or their communities;
- development of an emergency contact list to be included in the client/patient record for easy access in the case of emergency;
- assessment of technology issues for safety planning; and
- a plan to review safety plans and expectations with clients/patients (safety plans are the written steps for carrying out safety procedures and emergency protocols define the steps to be followed during emergency situations).

TYPES OF SAFETY ISSUES

The primary safety issues that may be encountered during TMH are generally the same as those experienced in in-office settings. These risks may include harm to self or others, worsening of symptoms that may contribute to heightened risk (e.g., suicidal ideation), and medical emergencies that could occur during a TMH session. We discuss these in greater detail in the following paragraphs.

Behavioral Emergencies

Behavioral emergencies include threats to harm others that involve duty to warn, and worsening of clinical symptoms, such as those resulting in heightened suicide risk. They require immediate clinical intervention. Although these same risks are present during traditional in-office practice, telepractice introduces additional consideration when safety planning given the geographic separation between the clinician and the client/patient. Effective TMH requires awareness of local emergency services as well as how far the client/patient may be from emergency or other help services in their community. The clinician should also know the average response time of police, fire, and other emergency services in all local areas where clients/patients are seen.

When TMH services are delivered to clinically supervised settings (i.e., hospitals or outpatient clinics), there will typically be on-site clinical staff available to assist and help resolve safety issues. TMH care delivered to an unsupervised setting requires additional planning steps because such staff are not involved. For example, a client/patient could indicate intent to harm himself or herself or another person at the end of a TMH session or while intentionally disconnecting the VC session. These types of situations require the TMH clinician to contact other identified support persons and/or law enforcement to assist at the client/patient's site.

Medical Emergencies

Medical emergencies present another risk, especially with homebound patients and patients with multiple chronic conditions. Behavioral medicine/health psychology services to unsupervised home settings may be particularly appealing to homebound individuals with serious conditions because of travel limitations and need for specific expertise. As these services expand, telepractitioners need to consider risks related to medical emergencies. For example, a client/patient could suffer cardiac arrest during a session and require notification of emergency services at the client/patient's location. Similarly, a client/patient may disclose to the telepractitioner that he or she had a recent fall or other injury in the home setting, yet had not self-identified the need to seek medical attention or was hesitant because of other barriers. The telepractitioner may provide additional support in completing the same steps the client/patient would follow if a medical emergency occurred separate from the telepractice session.

Risks Associated With Firearms

Access to firearms is another potential safety issue that teleproviders should consider, learning the social norms of the local community ahead of telepractice. ATA (Grady et al., 2011; Turvey et al., 2013) and APA (2013a) TMH guidelines state that clinicians shall discuss firearm ownership, safety, and the culture of firearms in rural areas. Access to firearms may be more of an imminent issue during home-based TMH and is a particular risk if a client/patient is known to have history of self-directed or other-directed violent behavior. Access to firearms should thus be taken into account when assessing the appropriateness of home-based TMH for some patients. However, as Pruitt, Luxton, and Shore (2014) noted, home-based TMH may be a safer alternative than in-office services when a patient has a history of violence or threatened violence toward clinical staff.

Many people who live in rural areas where hunting is common may have firearms in the home. When providing telepractice services with at-risk youth, teleproviders should be aware that it is common for a child may have knowledge of both the location of firearms and location of keys or lock combinations associated with access to ammunition, and also that parents may be unaware of the child's knowledge. Documentation of discussion and planning with children and parents about removal and/or safe storage of firearms in risky situations is important in the telepractice setting. Discussion of firearm access, regardless of setting, when safety is a concern is recommended. Furthermore, discussion of trigger safety lock devices may provide an additional level of safety precaution by restricting immediate access to firearms (Luxton, O'Brien, et al., 2012).

Risks Associated With Technical Difficulties

Technical problems with telehealth equipment (e.g., computers, monitors, video cameras, audio equipment) or network problems that cause a loss of connection may occur during a critical assessment or crisis situation and thus require an alternate method to contact the client/patient. Technology limitations, such as inadequate bandwidth for videoconferencing communication, insufficient camera resolution, or environmental problems (e.g., adequacy of room lighting and size, background noise or interruptions, room privacy, microphone placement) can also present a safety issue if audio/visual quality is impaired (Luxton, O'Brien, et al., 2012).

In some settings, VC equipment (e.g., laptop, camera or videophone) may be supplied by a care provider and therefore affords a level of control over the technical functioning of the equipment. However, the previously mentioned issues may especially be a risk during home-based TMH because of the potential disadvantage of relying on the network limitations of the patient's location as well as the patient's (or another family member's) personally owned equipment.

Not only should TMH providers have a secondary method for immediately contacting the patient and staff at the originating site in case of equipment failure, but they also should discuss with the patient up front what both parties will do in the event of technical malfunction. For instance, the practitioner may suggest that the client/patient remain off the telephone line so the clinician's efforts to call the client/patient will be successful. Such agreements can be made and documented as part of the informed consent process.

A patient or family in an unstable living situation, such as those going between living situations and homelessness, may not be the best fit for home-based telepractice because of difficulties in finding a consistent secure physical and technical environment to complete sessions. A similar discussion should occur if the client/patient connects from many different sites because of travel; assessment of whether travel locations will have adequate connectivity and environment to support telepractice sessions should be discussed.

CLIENT/PATIENT APPROPRIATENESS FOR TMH

An essential step is to assess whether providing TMH services is appropriate for each client/patient's circumstance. When patient records are available, it is good practice to review for history of adverse interactions during care, including violence toward family members or health care providers. Assessment of suicide risk prior to initiating and during treatment is also important (Luxton, O'Brien, Pruitt, Johnson, & Kramer, 2014). With the patient's consent, it is advisable to consult with other health care professionals who have been directly involved with treatment of the patient, such as referring providers. As with in-person settings, the individual's or family's preferences need to be taken into account and coercion avoided. For example, a clinician may recommend couple's therapy via a video conferencing platform, but one of the members of the couple may prefer telephone, in-person, or no services. Similarly, a school-based site may recommend TMH services but a parent/guardian may choose to refuse such treatment options for his or her child. In fact, giving priority to client/patient preference regarding TMH services is required by most professional association ethics codes and guidelines (ACA, 2014; APA, 2013a).

Along these lines, it is important to be mindful that clinical contraindications may be discovered during the course of clinical TMH services. At a minimum, telepractitioners should ask clients/patients on intake if they know of any issues that may present a barrier to participation in TMH, such as problems with vision or hearing that may limit the ability of patients to use VC equipment. In some situations, the VC setting may assist with such challenges, such as the ability for an individual with hearing impairment to zoom in on the clinician's face to read lips. It is important to make sure that the VC setting is easily accessible to patients across mobility and other health challenges.

In some situations, a client/patient with a history of adverse reactions to treatment may not be suitable for TMH care, particularly in unsupervised settings. For example, working with individuals struggling with serious anger management may call for extra caution on the part of the clinician when a client/patient is volatile and vulnerable people are also in the home. Once a client/patient is agitated in a nonclinical environment, it may be impossible for a telepractitioner to intervene effectively to calm the person before he or she interacts with others in the immediate environment. Telepractice sessions differ from in-person sessions in that the client/patient may have different exposure to family members and possibly less opportunity to decompress or "cool down" before heading home. In addition, both supervised and unsupervised TMH settings may have less access to on-site security personnel than in large in-person clinics.

Depending on the situation, clients/patients may require additional time to regain their composure, outside of what is normally allotted for their therapy session. For example, "Amy" was receiving therapy to learn to control her anger and anxiety, especially when dealing with her children. She told her therapist during their videoconference session that her goal was for all the children in her family—from her 20-year-old student to her 3-year-old niece she cared for during the week— to take part in keeping the house clean. While describing this goal, Amy became surprisingly agitated. Her therapist could hear the 3-year-old knocking on the door to Amy's room and calling for her aunt. It was easy to see how her niece's behavior was disruptive to Amy, and how difficult it was for Amy to remain in control of herself. In a situation such as this one, the telepractitioner can ask the patient to calm herself before addressing the children in question and to perhaps take a walk outside before speaking to anyone. In some cases, however, such a suggestion may not be heeded. If good diagnostic workups and related agreements are not in place, telepractitioners may find themselves at a crossroads with the need to make difficult choices about continuing or discontinuing care.

Telepractitioners should take additional safety precautions when working with victims of domestic violence in the home setting by ensuring that the abuser is not lurking out of the camera view. Similarly, child therapists should carefully assess safety in home environments if there is family history of interpersonal violence or if the presenting concern involves a family member (e.g., parent, sibling, other) bullying the child.

It is also common practice to develop verbal signals or code words to be used by the client/patient if something is amiss and the session needs to be terminated without any further verbal exchange. Another commonly used strategy, with the client's knowledge and consent, is for the clinician to scan the room with the camera to show the client/patient that no one else is in the room and to show the locked door. Likewise, the client/patient is then asked to do the same at his or her end of the connection, allowing the client/patient to tell potential lurkers that such scanning is commonplace.

Furthermore, clinicians carefully evaluate clients/patients with substance or alcohol abuse issues. Supervised settings providing these services may consider having breathalyzers or other screening tools available and training telepresenters to administer them. These patients may not be appropriate candidates to be seen in the home setting as clients/patients may have easier access to substances or alcohol in the home or may be more likely to use before or after a session. It also may be more difficult for clinicians to detect intoxication over video because they are not able to smell alcohol on the breath and may be less able to detect changes in voice amplitude, gait, etc. When working with any clinical population, the patient's engagement in a variety of addictive behaviors, including overeating, drinking, drugging, as well as excessive shopping and sexuality may need to be anticipated and addressed quickly by evoking a predefined protocol. Making it a point to explicitly ask patients about behaviors, such as whether they were drinking during the day, is an important part of such a protocol. If a patient endorses these behaviors, the patient and provider then follow the preestablished protocol, which in some cases may mean canceling that day's appointment or referring the patient for on-site services.

It is also important to assess the appropriateness of individuals interested in participating in group sessions over VC, particularly in unsupervised settings. Individuals with risk factors for suicidal concerns or decompensation are unlikely a good fit. Protocols for telepractice group sessions should include well-documented strategies to manage a participant should he or she decompensate within a video session or monopolize the encounter to the detriment of the other group members, including expectations to stop a session in the event a group member requires one-on-one support or direction to emergency services. Protocols, with associated informed consent processes, should describe how the telepractitioner will follow up with the individual and the other group members should a session be terminated. As in on-site settings, ground rules should be established concerning expectation for the privacy/security of the group sessions over video, as well as expectations for therapist and group member contact outside of sessions.

HOW TO DEVELOP A SAFETY PLAN

As a prerequisite, familiarity with the guidelines and ethics codes of applicable professional organizations is recommended. As outlined in Chapter 3, it is crucial for telepractitioners to be familiar with the jurisdictional requirements of the originating site. Some states have laws specific to telemedicine, and these laws vary from state to state in what type and under what circumstances care can be provided across state lines. It is necessary to be familiar with originating site civil commitment requirements as well as with duty-to-warn/protect requirements. Telepractitioners should also be aware of institutional-level guidance and protocols that may address these issues.

Ideally, safety planning is an ongoing process initiated in advance of difficulties, with protocols/procedures continuously revised as part of practice improvement processes. As in the face-to-face setting, strong team communication skills are crucial in developing and implementing safety plans. Some organizations, such as the U.S. Department of Veterans Affairs, have established standard operating procedures that include safety planning. Practitioners in private practice, however, may not have established safety protocols and thus must develop their own well-considered and written plans.

Review Safety Plans and Expectations With Clients/Patients

It is important for clinicians to discuss safety planning with clients/patients before initiating telepractice sessions as part of the informed consent process (APA, 2013a). The discussion of applicable confidentiality, data security (encryption/Health Insurance Portability and Accountability Act of 1996

[HIPAA] requirements), privacy, and safety procedures as they pertain to the home-based treatment is recommended. The roles and responsibilities of local collaborators, both lay supporters and health care professionals (e.g., telemedicine coordinators/presenters, medical teams), must be clearly defined in writing. In addition, full discussion and documentation of emergency procedures with appropriate family members or other identified local collaborators is advised (see Chapter 3). A setup session that includes such education may be needed prior to the initiation of treatment. When preparing for handling behavioral emergencies, a good diagnostic workup is essential to understanding how to best proceed.

Include Support People

With a solid informed consent agreement in place, the clinician is free to get to know local emergency processes, the availability of collateral services, and response times. The identification and use of a local collaborator, such as a family member or patient's friend, should also be considered as part of home-based TMH safety planning (APA, 2013a; Luxton, O'Brien, et al., 2012; Turvey et al., 2013). Community health workers also have potential to support patients in the home setting (see Chapter 9). Local health care professionals may also be able to provide technical assistance in the event that a connection is lost and, when appropriate, provide support to a client/patient in the event of emergency situations. However, telepractitioners must also remain sensitive to potential tensions in small communities when local supporters (e.g., family, friends, community health workers, health care professionals) become involved.

In some unsupervised VC situations, it may also make sense to consider collaborating with a second local care provider to help with care coordination in the event of psychiatric crises. Relationships and safety plans for clients/patients can be jointly developed with the cooperation of the local care provider to help handle emergencies.

Similarly, when working with people struggling with personality disorders or substance abuse, for example, it often is optimal to involve a team of local community professionals in the care plan, even when practicing in one's own professional community. This well-considered network of local care providers not only improves care by enhancing care coordination, but also minimizes risk and the practitioner's own anxiety when working with difficult patients. Establishing these relationships between the clinician and professionals in the client/patient's local community is also wise. These collateral services potentially involve not only the range of behavioral health and medical/nursing professionals, but also substance abuse treatment professionals, teachers, allied health professionals (e.g., physical therapists, speech therapists, occupational therapists), and a host of other professionals. Telepractitioners should also consider the risks of involving local collaborators in emergency situations (Luxton, O'Brien, et al., 2012). In particular, the safety of local collaborators must be carefully considered when managing crisis situations. If there is a safety risk to local collaborators, it may be best to rely on local emergency (911) responders. Telepractitioners should weigh the risks of disclosures made during emergency management on patient confidentiality and relationships, especially in small communities (Turvey et al., 2013). Although not always necessary, a physical visit to the community to identify and develop working relationships with local emergency personnel is optimal and, again, can build the local referral base.

ASSESSMENT FACTORS TO BE CONSIDERED AT A REMOTE SITE

Visiting the physical location and getting to know community resources at the remote site prior to engaging with a client/patient is often disregarded by online practitioners, but such relationship building is one of the best risk-management procedures and practice development strategies available (see Chapter 4). Rather than "shotgunning" services to many different communities online, it is suggested, then, that the practitioner identify several key communities to work and thereafter develop referral networks within those communities from which to give and receive referrals. By doing so, telepractitioners mirror traditional therapeutic involvement with community referral sources.

The purpose of such visits is to assess whether the TMH services fit local need. Listening and relationship building are the focus of these early meetings, allowing the community and future referrers to "put a name with a face," to get a better idea of the scope of TMH services, and to allay potential misperceptions regarding TMH. In many cases, it may allay community fears by clarifying that the telepractice service will fill service gaps, not compete with locally available services. Because many underserved communities have experienced few or no behavioral health providers in the past, few options for providers trained in the latest evidence-based practices, and/or high turnover among the behavioral providers, they may be cautious in embracing the new outreach service. It is advisable to take time in developing the telepractice and to avoid overpromising regarding scope of services (Nelson & Velasquez, 2011). For example, full implementation of telepractice from idea to full clinics often takes 1 to 2 years. It is important to maintain a dialogue with the community about a feasible time frame for the telepractice, often starting with a handful of patients to continuously improve processes ahead of ramping up to full capacity (see Chapter 4). Visits also assist with narrowing the scope of potential services, avoiding duplication of services, and building a referral network. Moreover, the visit and follow-up communication support the development of safety protocols by identifying the community-specific first responders and others who may assist in emergencies. For example, in developing a rural college telepractice, it is important to reach out to campus security services to discuss risk management concerns and procedures.

Particularly in rural areas, primary care providers may be de facto mental health services because of extreme referral shortages as well as the high prevalence of behavioral health conditions among primary care patients, and they are often important partners to cultivate when initiating telepractice. As many primary care practices are pursing patient-centered medical home designation, there is increasing interest in technologies to help coordinate care with behavioral health (Goldstein & Myers, 2014). Periodic visits (every 6 to 12 months) over video and in person with primary care providers and other local leaders will continue to grow these important community connections. Meeting with clients/patients in person can also be valuable. Some providers engage with communities by participating in cultural traditions, such as visiting a sweat lodge associated with rural American Indian veterans served by a TMH clinic (Shore et al., 2012).

As noted by Kramer, Mishkind, Luxton, and Shore (2013), emergency protocols should clearly delineate how two geographically distant sites will collaborate in technical, clinical/psychiatric, and medical emergencies. Ongoing protocol review and staff training are encouraged to support system/team readiness in the event of an emergency. In supervised TMH settings, protocols often take into account local emergency plans, as emergencies are generally handled consistent with already existing emergency protocols at the client/patient's site. Emergency plans should also clearly assign responsibility for contacting emergency and other necessary personnel (e.g., local law enforcement, facility security, emergency medical response teams). Both sites should have immediate access to emergency contact numbers that can respond to the originating (patient) site in the event of an emergency. Further, telepractitioners should obtain the direct phone number for emergency services for the location of patients and also test the nonemergency number for that area to verify that the emergency number is correct. Clinicians should also consider obtaining information regarding medical and psychiatric services that are nearby the patient to make appropriate referrals, to coordinate care across health care providers, and/or to contact the patient's medical team in the event of a crisis situation (Luxton, O'Brien, et al., 2012).

The following information should be collected and readily available to share with emergency personnel: the situation details, the patient's diagnosis and how it could influence interaction with law enforcement officers, and the contact information for local mental health support (Gros, Veronee, Strachan, Ruggiero, & Acierno, 2011; Luxton, O'Brien, et al., 2012; Maheu, Pulier, Wilhelm, McMenamin, & Brown-Connolly, 2004).

OPENING SESSION PROTOCOLS

Well-organized opening protocols for each session, including checklists, can establish the current location of the client/patient to ascertain compliance with legal and reimbursement requirements. Depending on the situation, room setup, locked doors, presence of other people in the room, child-care and eldercare arrangements, who if anyone (e.g., a nurse) is likely to see the patient record, possible interruptions, and other procedural issues should be reviewed. If it is learned that a client/patient is not in a location for which the clinician has collected required information, time can be taken at the beginning of that session to gather needed information before proceeding or to arrange for alternative care (e.g., reschedule for a later time) if the contact is deemed inappropriate—for example, a college student who is regularly seen over VC through her campus counseling office is visiting her parents for a holiday. Initial session discussion covered the location of her parents' home, location of local emergency resources, and the physical and technical environment. Of course, the clinical decision to see the patient in an alternate location is at the discretion of the practitioner and is based on professional judgment and client/patient condition at the time of each contact. When such decisions are made, the clinician is advised to carefully document rationales.

Uncertainty and fear of TMH, particularly home-based services, can be a barrier to improving access to care and meeting the needs of your clients/patients and the communities you serve. Again, remember that there is not any evidence that TMH, including home-based TMH, is less safe than in-office services when conducted according to evidence-based protocols. With knowledge of the risks, careful preparation, and practice, the TMH professional can ensure that the services they provide are delivered as safely and at the same level of quality as traditional in-office care.

6

Providing Direct Clinical Care

Telemental health (TMH) services that use videoconferencing (VC) have greatly expanded ways to provide quality clinical care across diverse general and underserved populations. Although clinical services via VC share many of the same considerations as traditional in-office services, providers must carefully consider the unique advantages and challenges of VC to assure optimal standards of care.

This chapter provides step-by-step guidance for conducting direct clinical services that include the range of behavioral health treatments with clients/patients. We specifically focus on setting up the clinical space and other telepractice preparation. We then summarize content and process components important to initial and follow-up telepractice sessions, as well as after-session components including documentation. If you are seeing clients/patients in a remote clinic environment, remember that the clinic will want to follow established protocols across preparation, initial

http://dx.doi.org/10.1037/14938-007
A Practitioner's Guide to Telemental Health: How to Conduct Legal, Ethical, and Evidence-Based Telepractice, by D. D. Luxton, E.-L. Nelson, and M. M. Maheu

sessions, and ongoing sessions, including protocol checklists to assist in monitoring areas of strengths and areas for improvement. If your practice primarily reaches individuals in their homes or other unsupervised setting, you must be cognizant of additional steps needed to safely and successfully deliver services to these settings. Remember that without clinical staff on-site, you will have to rely on your preestablished procedures for contacting local emergency services and/or a family member in an emergency. The integration of other technologies into the VC process will also be discussed, especially mobile devices and web-based applications. Although many of the same principles apply, Chapter 7 of this volume addresses best practices in psychological assessment and testing via TMH technologies.

SETTING UP THE TELEPRACTICE CLINICAL SPACE

It is good practice to consider both the client/patient's site(s) and the practitioner's site as clinical spaces. This includes both in formal clinical settings and when the services are provided directly to a client/patient's home. In a clinical setting, the space should accommodate the type of behavioral telehealth service provided; it should be large enough for the client/patient to feel comfortable during the encounter and possibly to allow the client/patient to demonstrate physical mobility, such as when conducting examinations. As in the on-site setting, a quiet room with comfortable furnishings fosters a welcoming, professional atmosphere at both the patient's and provider's location. With children and adolescents, it is often helpful to have a room that is large enough to accommodate a clinical staff person, the youth, and at least two other people (e.g., two parents/guardians, the parent and another child, or the parent and another person whom the parent might invite, such as a teacher). With younger children and other populations that may have limited attention, keep distractors in the remote clinic room to a minimum. As in the on-site setting, the TMH provider may set expectations at the beginning of sessions, such as not being able to continue a session if the child is under a table and out of the view of the camera. The materials provided and room size should accommodate evaluation of children's motor skills, play, and exploration, allowing the clinician to note atypical interactions or movements (Cain, Nelson, & Myers, 2015).

In the case of home-based services, the presence of roommates, family members, or pets, or unexpected phone calls and other distractions, may interrupt the encounter. It is therefore important for the TMH provider to work with the client/patient to schedule sessions during times that are as free of potential disruptions as possible. As part of informed consent and ongoing discussion, the client/patient should be discouraged from leaving the home environment with mobile VC (e.g., smartphone) and reminded not to drive or meet outside or in public places during the session. In the home setting, careful consideration should be given to patient appropriateness and establishing a safe telepractice environment, particularly when working with children. The TMH provider may choose not to see patients in the home if a previous abuser or bullier is in the same home environment because there is less provider control over whether this person may eavesdrop in the next room or potentially create a negative or unsafe environment. If a new disclosure of abuse is made during a home-based session, the teleprovider follows previously developed protocols and reminds the parent/guardian of the teleprovider's role as a mandated reporter (see Chapter 3). On the other hand, the home-based setting may be a particularly good fit in other situations with youth. For example, pediatric psychology services may be an option to support a child who is ill or whose guardian is homebound and who otherwise would struggle with transportation and other resources to attend sessions.

Both patient and clinician TMH spaces should be well lit, and the lighting in the room should be placed in a way that minimizes shadows and maximizes observing facial expression. If there are windows in the clinical space, they should have blinds or shades to both protect privacy and to control the amount of sunlight that is entering the room. Fluorescent lighting, especially soft or diffuse (i.e., nondirectional) light, is a good choice. Consider too that video cameras are sensitive to the amount of light and thus may create a poor image quality without adequate and evenly dispersed ambient light.

It is good practice to place the primary lighting source in front of a person rather than behind a person because back lighting can cause a shadow appearance. If overhead lighting is insufficient, you may consider asking the client/patient to find a lamp to put in front of his or her face. If the client/patient is to be seen in the home, a light commonly found on a coffee table or bed stand can often serve this purpose. Neutral, solid colors for the wall and the background of the room can also improve the picture quality. For the patients' benefit, it is also best for clinicians to keep the area within view of the camera clean and free from clutter or other potential visual distractions. For example, a messy bookcase, a bathrobe hung on the back of a door, or a cluttered laundry pile behind the clinician can convey the wrong impression, particularly when the patient is not able to scan the rest of the room to consider the context.

Cameras should be positioned in a way that allows the images of both parties to appear straight on and centered in their respective monitors so that both appear to speak eye to eye with each other. *Telepresence* or *eye-gaze angle* is the angle between the eye and the camera and the eye and the center of the display (Tam, Cafazzo, Seto, Salenieks, & Rossos, 2007). A potential problem when using VC technology is that users often make eye contact with the image of the person on the screen of their own computers rather than with the camera (Chen, 2002), which often can be located at the top edge of the computer monitor. This arrangement gives the appearance that one person is looking down or away from the other person. Eye contact between a client/patient and the clinician is important because it provides visual cues to which the participants can respond (Grayson & Monk, 2003; Maheu & McMenamin, 2004; Tam et al., 2007). Eye contact can be improved by attaching the camera to the central portion of the clinician's monitor (with duct tape, for instance) or by increasing the horizontal distance of participants from the VC unit. If the patient is using a mobile device for VC, it is important that the device is placed on a table or other secure surface so that a constant image can be maintained and holding the mobile device is not a distraction.

In addition, clients/patients may sometimes shift their position during a session, or the camera may be accidentally be bumped or moved from its optimal location. It may therefore be necessary to ask the patient to make adjustments before and during sessions. We have found that clients/patients often respond well to telepractitioners simply acknowledging this challenge with the technology and reinforce that they are giving full attention when not making full eye contact.

The picture-in-picture function available on many VC devices can be helpful to make sure that the provider is clearly in frame. It allows telepractitioners to see themselves as well as the clients/patient on their own monitors. For example, the clinician may not realize that his or her chair has shifted and the client/patient only sees half of the clinician's face and body. The PIP function may also be distracting, at least at first. Again, it is important to invite clients/patients to have an open dialogue about camera placement and other aspects of video quality throughout sessions and adjust the settings to match their preferences.

Technical problems that disrupt the VC connection may affect one end of the connection and not the other. Thus, it is good practice for clinicians to check in with clients/patients occasionally to make sure that they continue to see and hear clearly. It is also important to be mindful of how eye contact (eye gaze) when using VC may influence interactions during TMH. Taking notes or looking at other computer screens (e.g., to look at electronic health records) will disrupt eye contact. This has the potential to influence rapport as it will have the appearance that the clinician is distracted or disinterested. When taking notes or looking at medical records, it is good practice for clinicians to let clients/patients know what they are doing and why. Likewise, it may be useful for clinicians to give full permission to comment when they are inadvertently no longer fully on screen. It is prudent to ask clients/patients to speak freely about the clinician's lack of visibility or audibility or if the clinician is engaging in any behaviors that are distracting (e.g., tapping finger or pens, swiveling in the chair).

IN-SESSION CONSIDERATIONS

However odd some of these behaviors may seem, anecdotal complaints about telepractitioners have included such inappropriate behaviors as eating sandwiches or picking one's nose on camera, picking or licking teeth, filing or cleaning fingernails, cleaning one's ears, yawning repeatedly, and appearing in a bathrobe. Other clinicians have been reported doodling on notepads, tapping pens on desktops, twirling or rocking in their chairs, waving or shushing family members through glass windows or doors, yelling at dogs. Although most clinicians would never dream of voluntarily engaging in such activities in person, they apparently manage to convince themselves that others will not notice or mind such activities when on camera. It is prudent of the clinician to realize that cameras and microphones can be embarrassingly accurate and focus the patient's view to a very small part of the clinician's anatomy.

Telepractitioners should also consider other room-related features that may be apparent and modify them to create a welcoming, professional clinical space. They should be mindful of pictures on the wall and other room décor, consciously assessing whether this complements the intended professional atmosphere. Messy backgrounds with disorderly papers crammed into dusty bookshelves or clothes strewn on exercise equipment should be avoided.

The TMH clinician should consider the level of remote control that he or she needs of the distant camera. The clinician may control the camera and scan the room at the distant site to understand who is in the environment. In addition, and with the patient's permission, the clinician may elect to zoom in to assess important physical presentations such as tics, gait, or other relevant clinical features. If the clinician is tempted to use the distant camera to zoom in without asking for the patient's permission, it may be important to realize that some zooming cameras emit an audible sound.

It is also important to ensure that the audio is loud enough at each end so patient and provider can adequately hear each other without straining. Keep in mind that volumes should be comfortable and that if too loud, the session may be overheard by people outside the room or in adjacent rooms. People often speak louder when using VC, and speakers tend to have greater volume levels than the voice does during in-person sessions. A quiet room, located away from noisy hallways and clinic reception areas, is preferred. Simple solutions include posting a "Quiet Please" sign when the room is in use.

In noisier settings, it may help to install soundproofing material on ceilings and walls to reduce unwanted sound transmission and to ensure patient privacy. This can be especially true if the clinician's site is near bus routes or other busy traffic areas, including air traffic. Audio feedback is a common challenge during telepractice sessions; the technician can assist with practical solutions including adjusting volume at one or both sides as well as positioning speakers to decrease such feedback. Parents can assist children in avoiding playing with toys immediately next to microphones, as this may produce uncomfortable levels of noise.

VC camera systems may have trouble focusing when there is too much movement. Thus, practitioners should be mindful of physical movements (e.g., hand gestures) during VC sessions as these may be distracting to the client/patient and disruptive to the overall process. Clinicians may provide additional vocal acknowledgements as this can help assure that they can be heard and seen adequately.

SESSION PREPARATION

Before initiating clinical services, the provider establishes who will be seen and who is not a fit for his or her telepractice clinic, guided by individual preference and clinical strengths; research and telepractice guidelines; and institutional policies (see also the discussion of patient appropriateness in Chapter 5). With children, these considerations include the child's presenting concern and developmental level, the parents' preferences, the resources at the distant/presenting side, and the provider's comfort level (Myers, Cain, & Work Group, 2008). Similarly, the clinician decides which clients/patients will be seen in person for initial interviews and which will be seen over VC for the initial clinical encounter; practices successfully function using both approaches. The telepractitioner is encouraged to consult legal counsel about current local, state, and federal laws that may impact guidance about seeing a patient first in person, particularly in the event that the teleprovider is prescribing scheduled medications.

Depending on the TMH clinic's scheduling process, clients/patients may first contact the provider or the distant site. As part of the scheduling process, the administrative personnel convey basic information about the telepractice setting and about the clinical services available.

Interested clients/patients are then sent paperwork associated with the telepractice clinic.

Although the paperwork varies by clinic and patient age, it often includes a behavioral intake form, behavior rating scales (across patient, family, school personnel, and/or other informants), consent to treatment form, the Notice of Privacy Practices associated with the Health Insurance Portability and Accountability Act of 1996 (HIPAA), and information concerning the patient's financial responsibilities with the clinic (e.g., a copy of the insurance card). Some information may be competed securely online; other copyrighted materials may be mailed. Completed paperwork should be sent following the organization's data management procedures, including mailing and faxing information when needed; organizational policy should be reviewed when considering e-mailing or sending digital images of information. Because TMH may focus on increasing access for underserved clients/patients, telepractitioners should consider the language, literacy, and health literacy needs of the target audience (see Chapter 9). The distant site coordinator often assists families new to behavioral health in addressing early questions and supporting paperwork completion.

The provider or the site coordinator provides initial information to inform the client/patient about whether telepractice may be a good option for his or her specific needs. For example, if driving to a clinic is an alternative option, the pros and cons should be discussed with the client/patient. Additionally, the provider and/or site coordinator may talk with interested individuals about their comfort and competence with the chosen technology before scheduling. A client/patient's familiarity and experience with any given technology may range from none to very experienced. The patient's experience and preferences regarding technology should be documented to be in compliance with some professional guidelines. Questions to ask may include the following:

- Have you ever received mental health services?
- If so, did you experience telemental health? What experiences have you had with technologies when working with a counselor or therapist? Were they positive or negative? Was anything particularly useful for you? Distracting or annoying?

- Do you have any experience with Skype or FaceTime?
- How comfortable are you with general technologies such as using the Internet, texting, or other technologies?

When connecting with a new site or a site with new staff and technologies, a test connection is strongly encouraged ahead of the appointment. This allows the technician to work with the telepractitioner, the site coordinator, and the patient/family to address concerns ahead of time and decrease anxieties on the day of the appointment. As detailed in Chapters 2 and 4, it is important to keep in mind that technology limitations, such as inadequate bandwidth, insufficient camera resolution, or environmental problems (e.g., adequacy of room lighting, microphone placement), may be especially an issue during home-based TMH because of reliance on the Internet connection at the client/patient's location and on the use of personally owned equipment (e.g., Internet Service Provider, webcams). Thus, an assessment of the available technology and specifications should be conducted prior to initiating treatment. Discussion of safety procedures and expectations is also a must (see Chapter 5 for detailed information). Specific attention should be given to discussion of policies and procedures for clinical emergencies as well as description of the roles of each party (provider, patient, and family site coordinator and staff at the remote site).

INITIATING AND CONDUCTING TELEPRACTICE SESSIONS

Initial telepractice sessions include the same key elements as initial on-site sessions, with the addition of telepractice information. The intake provides an opportunity for the client/patient to share what brought him or her to therapy, for the therapist to share initial clinical impressions and overall approach, and for both to talk together about whether the telepractice is a good fit to meet the goals. Telepractitioners often begin by introducing themselves and their services. Many clients are new to behavioral health, and these introductions help to demystify the therapy process and set expectations in working together toward a common goal. When applicable, the site coordinator's role in supporting the session is discussed, including expectations of when the site coordinator will be physically present and when how the site coordinator will be accessible when outside of the room, as well as assurances that the site coordinator is a health care professional who adheres to the same high level of confidentiality as the teleprovider. In child therapy for example, the site coordinator may direct individuals in going between the telepractice room and the waiting room as the telepractitioner talks individually with the child and then with the parent(s). Clients/patients may have preexisting expectations of the TMH process depending on previous experiences, if any. If, for example, they have had negative experiences with computer technology in the past (e.g., getting commercial VC software to work on their personal computer), they may worry about whether TMH will work for them. It may be necessary to reassure individuals who are apprehensive about TMH that there are processes in place to help sessions run smoothly and that they will be provided the support that they need to feel comfortable. If there continues to be unease about moving forward, the telepractitioner and the patient will jointly agree to terminate the VC session.

Because of the additional novelty added by technology, it is even more important than in on-site encounters to welcome client/patient questions and concerns throughout the telepractice sessions. This open dialogue facilitates client/patient comfort and builds rapport. Consider too that some clients/patients may be very experienced with technology and that leveraging a client/patient's technical experience in a collaborative way can also be very useful for establishing a working alliance (Pruitt, Luxton, & Shore, 2014).

As part of the intake, the telepractitioner discusses the same key components of consent to treatment (see Chapter 3) as completed on-site, with an emphasis on the client/patient's choice of whether to engage in the services. Components often include informing clients/patients about the therapy expectations and duration; attendance policies; explaining fees and payment policies; discussing the involvement of third parties; and reviewing the limits of confidentiality around safety concerns, mandated reporting requirements, and when applicable, status as a minor. Discussion about communication with the provider is reviewed, including after-hours contact as well as crisis management approaches. In addition, the telepractitioner provides information about data security, encryption technology, and limits of data use at the onset of clinical services. Although these should be covered in the informed consent process before initiating treatment (see Chapter 3 for informed consent procedures), it is also good practice to mention them again during the initial session. In home-based TMH, there may be other family members or guests in the patient's living environment. It is therefore good practice to ask clients/patients if they feel that their space is private and if they expect any disruptions during the session. Clients/patients should also be informed that the VC session is not being recorded. As with in-person care, most VC sessions are not recorded. A thorough explanation and documentation is needed if sessions are to be recorded for any reason.

The first session also includes a brief discussion of technical troubleshooting steps and procedures, including a user-friendly instruction sheet. This is particularly important in the home setting, where information is provided about who to call in the event of technical problems and step-by-step instructions for what to do if the VC connection is lost. It is a good idea to remind the clients/patients that you can see them, even when the audio is muted, and that they can see you throughout sessions. This is especially important for clients/patients who are new to VC technology or for group sessions in which the VC camera needs to be positioned to view all participants. Let clients/patients know who else is participating in the session on the provider side (e.g., other team members, trainees) and introduce each person. Ask the client/patient who is participating on his or her side (e.g., other family members, other persons involved in the care of the client/patient), as well as scan the room remotely when feasible to view those off camera.

Keep in mind that an initial TMH session may take longer than an in-office session because of the need to discuss extra steps such as technical troubleshooting and safety planning. If working without technical support, budget time accordingly to talk about behavioral services in general as well as technology-related questions. The telepractitioner and client/patient discuss whether telepractice is a match for the client/patient's needs. If it is a match, they discuss scheduling the next session and consider a time frame for therapy. If not a match, they may discuss other treatment options.

To deliver services matching the standard of care, telepractice sessions approximate the same content and process components as in-person behavioral services. This works best when the telepractitioner has had the opportunity to develop a strong comfort level with the technology through training, shadowing, mentoring, and practice (see Chapter 8). To start, clinicians may want to identify themselves and their location at the initiation of contact with a client/patient, then ask the client/patient to his or her identify and location. This exchange establishes the identity of both parties and their locations, which is helpful in documenting compliance with the requirement of having met the legal needs for licensure. This quick and simple protocol also helps identify the location of service for billing purposes when a third party payer is involved. This "opening protocol" can be elaborated to establish other professional aspects of the relationship, ask for security compliance, remind the client/patient of prior agreements, and so forth (Turvey et al., 2013).

Across initial and follow-up telepractice sessions, the telepractitioner carefully monitors the therapeutic alliance and notes shifts that may occur in rapport over the course of providing services. During sessions, telepractitioners closely attend to nonverbal reactions as they would in onsite sessions, including silences and body language. Facial expressions and reactions such as crying continue to be important information to guide telepractice process.

AFTER TELEPRACTICE SESSIONS

As in in-person sessions, it is good practice to conclude by asking clients/patients to share any further questions that they may have about the therapy process in general, as well as their experiences with the technology. The telepractitioner and the client/patient may discuss having in-person sessions or other options if the patient's needs or situation have changed. For example, if a patient endorses increased suicidal ideation and other manifestations of declining functioning, the patient and provider may agree to an in-person visit, at which time they can consider future telepractice sessions together. The telepractitioner and client/patient discuss scheduling the next session as well as recommendations, including referrals and homework. At sites using electronic health records, the telepractitioner may discuss the after-visit summary with the client/patient, including faxing or mailing per client/patient request. With the client/patient consent, the telepractitioner may provide a summary of recommendations to the site coordinator. For example, if the services are provided through the client/patient's medical network, a summary may be sent to the primary care provider with the consent of the client/patient.

In addition, the telepractitioner completes documentation requirements outlined in the telepractice protocol, using the same standards and methods as in-office care. It is important to document in the patient/client's records where both the originating and distant sites are located and that the behavioral health services were provided using VC technology (or other technology if used). Generally, the site where the patient is located should assure that all necessary preencounter documentation (e.g., intake and consent forms) is completed and securely transferred to the provider site for review. All record keeping, including the storage and transmission of patient records, should be done in accordance with local, state, and federal laws, including compliance with HIPAA requirements.

If the telepractice bills insurers, it is important to know how to use CPT (Current Procedural Terminology) codes to be reimbursed for TMH services. In general, the same behavioral health CPT codes (e.g., individual therapy, group therapy, health and behavior codes) that are used in on-site practice are used in the telepractice setting, with the addition of the general telemedicine modifier. Government insurance programs such as Medicare and Medicaid as well as third-party insurance companies use CPT codes to designate what health care services they will pay for and how much they will pay (more information at http://www.cms.gov/Outreach-and-Education/Medicare-Learning-Network-MLN/MLNProducts/downloads/TelehealthSrvcsfctsht.pdf). Telepractitioners should review the specific requirements of Medicare and their state's Medicaid program in relation to telehealth billing. The telepractitioner is encouraged to check with the individual insurers that are relevant to his or her practice about general telepractice coverage, as well as the specific codes covered in the telepractice setting. Be sure to check with your local institution's requirements related to reimbursement and documentation procedures.

INTEGRATING OTHER TECHNOLOGIES INTO CLINICAL CARE

There are other health technologies that may be integrated with VC services such as the use of home-monitoring devices, as well as smartphone and tablet apps and websites. These technologies expand the capabilities of telepractitioners and also provide clients/patients with useful self-help tools. For example, Internet websites can be used to share psychoeducational materials, provide assessments, connect patients into a support network, etc. Smartphone and tablet apps can be used for a variety of therapeutic purposes including self-help information or guidance, psycho-education, self-monitoring tools and adherence, and biofeedback. Mobile apps are available to address just about any topic including anxiety, depression, smoking, alcohol and substance use, cognitive performance, psychosis, diet, exercise, weight loss, nutrition, parenting, relationships, relaxation, sleep, spirituality, general well-being, and more (Luxton, McCann, Bush, Mishkind, & Reger, 2011). At the time of this writing, there is not a standardized certification process for apps or for what meets HIPAA compliance.

The use of these mobile health devices and apps may increase privacy risks given that data may be transmitted over unsecure wireless connections, or data stored with apps may be sent to unauthorized third parties (Luxton, Kayl, & Mishkind, 2012). An example might be someone who uploads a diary entry to an unprotected web server that subsequently gets hacked or personal information that one company shares with another company. Therefore all privacy and data security recommendations should be thoroughly investigated by the prescribing practitioner. Then, risks and expectations for use of these technologies should be disclosed and discussed during the informed consent process. It is also important to consider that the asynchronous aspect of some technologies, such as the Internet, e-mail, and SMS texting, and remind clients/patients of the duration of time that may elapse before they can expect to receive a response.

7

Conducting Psychological Assessments During Telemental Health

As with any new area of practice, the ethics of conducting assessment via technology requires specific experience, training, supervision, and consultation. Those requirements are paramount when shifting in-person assessment to online or other telehealth modalities. Telemental health (TMH) providers must consider how the test results will be used (e.g., for clinical assessment, symptom monitoring, data collection for research). Also, how will informed consent be completed? Does the administration of the assessment via technology have an impact on reliability and validity of test scores? Who will administer the assessment? How should the instrument be scored and interpreted? How will the results be explained to the client/patient and, with children, to the parent/guardian? How will the assessment protocol be followed and test security maintained? Finally, how will test data and evaluation results be shared with other professionals involved in the patient's care?

http://dx.doi.org/10.1037/14938-008
A Practitioner's Guide to Telemental Health: How to Conduct Legal, Ethical, and Evidence-Based Telepractice, by D. D. Luxton, E.-L. Nelson, and M. M. Maheu

The American Psychological Association (APA) provides general guidance about these processes and has included them in the *Ethical Principles of Psychologists and Code of Conduct* (APA, 2010a) and *Guidelines for the Practice of Telepsychology* (APA, 2013a). Other professional membership groups have published similar yet more global requirements for their professionals using assessment instruments online (American Counseling Association, 2014; Grady et al., 2011; National Association of Social Workers, 2008; Turvey et al., 2013). To deliver best practices, clinicians across disciplines are encouraged to stay current with the scientific literature as well as publications on assessment by professional associations and TMH-focused organizations.

In this chapter, we provide the practitioner with an overview of the best methods for conducting clinical assessments across distance with technologies. This includes selecting measures/tests, ensuring optimal assessment conditions and procedures when using telehealth technologies, and applying best practices for administering assessments remotely.

REMOTE ASSESSMENT METHODS AND BENEFITS

The benefits of remote assessment can perhaps be best understood in light of an example. Let's take the case of a disruptive teenager who abuses multiple substances and who has just been arrested by the local police for verbally threatening an officer. The court would seek rapid, reliable information to support decision making around the youth's placement and consequences. Remote assessment would include a thorough clinical interview over videoconferencing (VC) conducted by a pediatric psychologist specializing in juvenile forensics, as well as validated assessment questionnaires completed online. In this case, both depression and substance abuse could be diagnosed, which ultimately could support the court's decision to mandate residential treatment for the teen. As in traditional clinic settings, this case highlights the importance of using a variety of information sources to make diagnoses and recommendations, in tandem with clinical interview and observation. Clinical interviews, whether conducted in person or with VC, provide more information about the patient than is possible with a survey instrument alone.

All assessment approaches have advantages and disadvantages. The professional balances quality, access, and patient safety when selecting the best assessment battery and administration methodology. Methods can include traditional telephones for synchronous (real-time) communication as well as asynchronous (store-and-forward) technologies such as e-mail and fax to send and receive assessment materials. The Internet can also be used to administer psychological tests and measurements remotely on web pages, with several advantages over the use of paper-and-pencil questionnaires. In general, online assessments are less time-consuming and less costly, and they can be distributed more easily to large populations. Online data entry is automated and therefore less sensitive to human error in entry, and there is less risk of missing data (Kongsved, Basnov, Holm-Christensen, & Hjollund, 2007). Research in some areas of assessment has suggested decreased impact of social desirability when completing surveys online, as well as greater self-disclosure in some populations (Joinson, 1999). The telepractitioner should also be aware of limitations, including the negative impact of slow or terminated Internet connection and variable questionnaire appearance based on screen size and screen resolution (Bartram, 2006).

Smart mobile devices (i.e., smartphones and tablets) have become an important addition to the diagnostician's toolbox to more efficiently and accurately conduct assessments. For instance, mood and anxiety measures can now be in the form of an application or "app" on mobile devices or accessed via Internet with data uploaded for easy clinician review (Luxton, McCann, Bush, Mishkind, & Reger, 2011). Assessment apps on smart mobile devices can be useful for measuring the dynamic characteristics of a person. For instance, subjective mood or anxiety levels can be tracked in real time or data from biofeedback equipment can be tracked and analyzed remotely. Emerging approaches use a range of mobile technology capabilities (e.g., sensors, GPS) to assist in evaluating and predicting needs for support in depression and many other conditions (Burns et al., 2011; Luxton et al., 2011). However, clinicians should also be aware of risks associated with the broad availability of online and mobile-based self-screening measures. For example, one of the authors has had a patient present with concern after scoring "depressed" using the app version of a mood ring. We recommend that clinicians ask their clients/patients about what health-related apps they may be using and review available information about any app of interest to assess the overall quality and appropriateness (Luxton, June, & Chalker, 2015).

LEGAL, POLICY AND PRACTICE STANDARDS REVIEW

When considering the need for conducting remote clinical assessments, the initial step is a policy and practice standards review. This includes a comprehensive review of current laws and policies in the jurisdiction and setting of practice (see Chapter 3, this volume). The telepractitioner should assess his or her competence in the assessment approach, in delivering feedback, and in using the technology. If gaps are noted, the telepractitioner follows up with additional training/mentoring as needed. TMH practitioners need to know best practices regarding when to use an assessment instrument, which types of psychological assessments or tests are appropriate, and which settings require adaptations or are inappropriate.

In some settings, in-person psychological assessments may be the standard of care and the only option. In other settings, however, an in-person assessment may be required at first contact with patients, and subsequent assessments may then be accomplished remotely. In the United States, the Centers for Medicare and Medicaid Services (CMS) have approved Current Procedural Terminology (CPT) code sets related to technology-based assessment (see http://www.cms.gov/Outreach-and-Education/Medicare-Learning-Network-MLN/MLNProducts/downloads/TelehealthSrvcsfctsht.pdf). Furthermore, the 2015 Medicare Physician Fee Schedule Final Rule (October 1, 2014), effective January 1, 2015, states the following:

> CPT codes 96103 (psychological testing (includes psychodiagnostic assessment of emotionality, intellectual abilities, personality and psychopathology, e.g., MMPI), administered by a computer, with qualified health care professional interpretation and report); and, 96120 (neuropsychological testing (e.g., Wisconsin Card Sorting Test), administered by a computer, with qualified health care professional interpretation and report). These services involve testing by computer, can

> be furnished remotely without the patient being present, and are payable in the CMS-1612-FC 194 same way as other physicians' services. These remote services are not Medicare telehealth services as defined under the Act; therefore, we need not consider them for addition to the telehealth list, and the restrictions that apply to telehealth services do not apply to these services.

Practitioners conducting psychological assessments with telehealth technology also need to be cognizant of all relevant laws for all jurisdictions served. In the United States, this includes the Health Insurance Portability and Accountability Act of 1996 (HIPAA), the Health Information Technology for Economic and Clinical Health Act, applicable federal and state laws, and local privacy and security requirements. In Canada, federal laws include the Personal Information Protection and Electronic Documents Act. Almost all countries now have legal requirements for using not only the Internet, but also a wide array of technologies.

The American Telemedicine Association provides specific practice standards and guidelines regarding legal review (Grady et al., 2011; Turvey et al., 2013). Appropriate disclosure of safeguards and potential risks associated with privacy and electronic data should be addressed during the informed consent process. However, as pointed out by Maheu and McMenamin (2013), the informed consent process or an agreement with patients may not be adequate in all situations, in all states, or in foreign countries. The same can be expected in other countries. The clinician then, must be aware of such laws, understand them, and be in full compliance to be administering assessments across state and national borders. Moreover, the diversity in the types of technologies, network infrastructures, and procedures for their use requires careful review of data security risks and requirements (see Kramer, Mishkind, Luxton, & Shore, 2013; Luxton, Kayl, & Mishkind, 2012).

A related example might involve a copyrighted psychological questionnaire. If such an instrument is used as part of assessment, the publisher's rules concerning the sharing of the instrument online must be closely followed. In many instances, the instrument may need to be mailed to the client/patient for completion and then mailed back to the telepractitioner for scoring. Very specific instructions may need to be included to maintain the standardization of test administration, as dictated by various professional association ethical standards (see Ethical Standards related to assessment; APA, 2010a).

CLIENT/PATIENT SPECIFIC VARIABLES

Ethical and competent assessment practice requires careful consideration and awareness of many client/patient specific variables. As stated in the APA's (2013a) *Guidelines for the Practice of Telepsychology*, psychologists are expected to consider geographic location, technological competence (both psychologist and client/patient), medical conditions, mental status and stability, psychiatric diagnosis, current or historic use of substances, treatment history, and therapeutic needs that may be relevant to assessing the appropriateness of the services offered. It would be reasonable for other types of professionals to adhere to similar guidelines and to have these issues addressed when using any type of remote psychological assessment.

Prior to engaging in remote assessments, it is wise to review the patient's clinical history to determine potential clinical, cognitive, and/or sensory deficits that could impair his or her ability to use telehealth technology. If remote assessment is expected to be difficult for a client/patient who is visually impaired or has hearing difficulties, in-person assessment may be recommended. Technological aids (e.g., headsets, screen magnification devices, speech-to-text translation software) or the assistance of family members or other caregivers and local collaborators (see Chapter 5) may be appropriate. Possible fatigue or physical discomfort caused by technology use (e.g., eye strain when viewing computer monitors) should also be evaluated before and during the assessment process, especially during lengthy assessment sessions (Luxton, Pruitt, & Osenbach, 2014).

Individual backgrounds may also present a strong contextual influence on whether and how technology is used with specific cultures (Brooks, Spargo, Yellowlees, O'Neill, & Shore, 2012; see also Chapter 9, this volume). It is also important for practitioners to be sensitive to the capabilities and preferences of clients/patients during assessments. For example, some clients/patients may have very little experience with technology and thus may be apprehensive or less engaged during a TMH-based assessment.

On the other hand, some clients/patients may appreciate the additional personal space afforded through the technology and prefer TMH-based assessment. It is best to ask the individual patient about technology interest and preferences, avoiding assumptions based on age or other characteristics. Also, examiners may need clients/patients to take a basic language comprehension test to assess language skills when working remotely. Such language comprehension tests are available online and assess both spoken and written English. Health literacy evaluation may also be indicated.

SAFETY CONSIDERATIONS

Safety is the priority for telepractitioners during TMH assessments. In general, the same safety planning presented in Chapter 5 should be followed with all remote assessments. For example, there should be a predefined safety plan if a client/patient becomes distressed or has a medical emergency during a remote assessment session. When using online assessment tools that include items about suicide/homicide, it is important to have strategies in place that allow quick clinician response should a client/patient report high risk. Therefore, patients with a history of adverse reactions to treatment (e.g., severe panic attacks), or those who are at high risk of harm to self or others (e.g., family members in the case of home-based TMH), may not be appropriate for telehealth-based assessment (Luxton, O'Brien, McCann, & Mishkind, 2012). Clinicians should consider the pros and cons of continuing the assessment and, as with any conventional in-person assessment, document and disclose how those factors may have influenced assessment results (Luxton, Pruitt, & Osenbach, 2014). Similarly, the safety of the client/patient and family members must be considered when conducting remote assessments and giving results from a distance.

SELECTING APPROPRIATE ASSESSMENT MEASURES AND TECHNIQUES

Just as in on-site practice, telepractitioners must familiarize themselves with the available scientific literature regarding a measure or technique's appropriateness for the intended use, as well as its reliability and validity

(Luxton, Pruitt, & Osenbach, 2014). Test selection should be guided by research and clinical expertise, with careful consideration of what the provider would anticipate to be better, the same, or worse with technology-based administration. Of particular importance are multicultural, multilingual, and other diversity issues and an instrument's validity and reliability with the populations being assessed (see Chapter 9).

The evidence examining the psychometric properties of telehealth-based assessments is growing, yet there are gaps in the literature that practitioners should consider when selecting assessment instruments and mediums. Professionals administering tests in alternative environments need to consider that the majority of available measures and assessment tools are based on norms established for in-person assessment. Extrapolation to administration through one or more telecommunication mediums may be inappropriate. For instance, a Patient Health Questionnaire (PHQ-9) delivered in-person or by web page versus over the telephone can yield substantially different results depending on technology chosen (Turvey, Willyard, Hickman, Klein, & Kukoyi, 2007). Also, mobile devices vary in the size and quality of their display screens and therefore do not necessarily present information similarly. Thoughtful consideration should be given concerning what, if any, reasons the provider might have that would lead him or her to anticipate different results over a technology medium. Although still early, published reviews regarding the psychometric properties of psychological and cognitive functioning assessments conducted via telehealth technologies are beginning to surface in the evidence base (see Backhaus et al., 2012; Grady et al., 2011; Luxton, Pruitt, & Osenbach, 2014). Expert consultation with assessment tool developers/leaders and experienced telepractitioners may be helpful. In all cases, careful review of the instructions or administration manuals should be conducted to determine appropriateness.

Optimizing the Assessment Setting

In some ways, the TMH clinician will have less control over the remote setting than would be possible during in-office setting. The telepractitioner and, when applicable, the distant site coordinator/presenter strive to assure that the environmental conditions are favorable to assessment procedures (see Chapter 6). Through the informed consent process, the clinician is transparent about his or her role and the intended use of the assessment information. For example, if the clinician is completing a psychological or other evaluation in a forensic role, then this should be articulated and documented. If the clinician is completing an assessment as a school consultant, the intended use of the evaluation by the school should be clearly delineated and understood. Information about the length of the session(s), the number of anticipated sessions, opportunities for breaks (if applicable), and the plan to share the findings with the client/patient and others should be disclosed.

In general, the room at the distant location should be large enough to be comfortable, should be well lit, and should have sound levels adjusted (for more information, see Chapter 6). Assessments that involve group or family interviews will require a space that is large enough to accommodate the group. Some applications may require the addition of a table and other supplies. Multiple cameras may also be optimal, so as to see the family's actions from multiple angles concurrently. With the direction of the clinician, the telemedicine coordinator/presenter may assist with managing who is in and outside of the room. In home-based assessment, the presence of family members, roommates, pets, or unexpected visitors as well as phone calls may be disruptive. It is thus important to adjust scheduling to minimize disruptions.

In situations in which a feedback session is completed over VC, the approach mirrors traditional on-site approaches to assessment feedback. If reviewing a written report is integral, the clinician may consider strategies to transmit the report to the client/patient ahead of time, if clinically appropriate, as well as providing a signed copy of the results. Because VC is often used to provide services in underserved communities, it may be challenging to identify resources to support recommendations, and the clinician may need to budget additional time to talk with the client/patient and caregiver about treatment strategies. With the consent of the client/patient and caregiver, some feedback sessions may include a local support team, such as a spouse, home health nurse, teacher, primary care provider, or others. Emerging models use technology to link multiple systems of care to enhance the assessment process. For example, R. M. Reese et al. (2015) described a cost-effective integrated system using a telemedicine model for autism evaluation. Using real-time VC, this model links families, trained early intervention providers and educators at remote sites, and an interprofessional diagnostic team at the academic health center.

Technology-Specific Considerations

The telepractitioner and, when applicable, distant site coordinator/presenter and staff also consider the client/patient's ability to assess and respond to nonverbal communication. Nonverbal information is useful for determining the patient's emotional state and, in some cases, high-risk or other nonverbal behaviors that are indicative of emotional states worthy of attention. For example, body posture, facial expressions, body language (e.g., foot tapping, hand wringing), facial flushing, tearing up, and direction of eye gaze, may provide important information. Psychomotor functioning and other medical symptoms are also necessary to observe during psychological assessments. VC assessments may be influenced by camera angle, screen size, room characteristics, or other technical factors (e.g., network bandwidth issues) that make it difficult to view all of the client/patient's behaviors.

In unsupervised settings such as the home, the lack of in-person physical presence may limit the range of information available. In supervised TMH settings, it can be important to maximize the site coordinator's assistance as the provider's "eyes and ears" at the site, as well as in asking clarifying questions. For example, the site coordinator may detect alcohol on the client or caregiver's breath or hygiene concerns. Because of often long-standing relationships between the site coordinators and the clients/patients, they may help detect subtle changes in the client/patient behavior as well, such as when a patient is shaken by the test results and might be a danger to himself or herself as a result.

Given the potential limits of what and how information can be collected during remote assessments, it may be appropriate to modify procedures. For instance, it may be necessary to ask a patient to hold a paper-and-pencil assessment (e.g., self-report measures or therapy homework) up to the video camera for viewing or to use larger handwriting because of small screen size or poor image quality. In addition, it may be helpful to ask the client/patient to read responses out loud in scenarios in which video is not used or when the connection quality is less than optimal. When nonverbal information is unavailable or limited, additional questions may be needed to improve the accuracy.

Other Considerations

A general search of the Internet will reveal many types of published psychological tests available online. The reader is cautioned, as their availability does not qualify all assessments labeled as such as appropriate tests for licensed professionals to use with a worldwide population. Any assessment's intended audience, design, and security of processes are essential factors to be considered by the professional. TMH practitioners also need to consider whether remote administration of assessment materials presents a risk to the integrity of the instrument (e.g., by clients/patients being able to print items at home or share them via social media). Practitioners should also consider whether there is an increased risk for dishonest responses (e.g., responses obtained from the Internet or someone else taking the assessment) because control over the testing environment is reduced (Buchanan, Johnson, & Goldberg, 2005; Reips, 2000). A good litmus test for the appropriateness of a test for any given population is to check with the test publisher to ascertain that its digitized availability is authorized. Report any unauthorized use of copyrighted testing material if found.

Also, those professionals working with technology development companies share an even greater responsibility because promoting the use of online assessments without sufficient data or with inappropriate methods could be considered a conflict of interest and a violation of ethical standards. Furthermore, the reevaluation of these assessment tools with diverse populations, clinical presentations, and telehealth technologies is necessary to assure the validity of assessments conducted via technology of any kind.

8

Telesupervision and Training in Telepractice

Videoconferencing-based supervision, or *telesupervision*, involves a trainee at one site securely videoconferencing (VC) with a supervisor at another site. For example, clinicians training in small communities may benefit from additional supervision reflecting different expertise and decreased likelihood of multiple relationships. In addition, trainees may seek training in very specialized areas in which there are only a handful of national experts. Others who live in remote areas where there is limited or not any access to clinical experts in specialty behavioral health areas may benefit from "teleconsultation" whereby professionals consult with colleagues at a distance to receive clinical and professional guidance. Furthermore, behavioral health clinicians, particularly those who work by themselves in private practice, can experience feelings of isolation and burnout. Supervision and consultation via VC can also help address these issues (R. J. Reese et al., 2009).

http://dx.doi.org/10.1037/14938-009
A Practitioner's Guide to Telemental Health: How to Conduct Legal, Ethical, and Evidence-Based Telepractice, by D. D. Luxton, E.-L. Nelson, and M. M. Maheu

Telesupervision has supported individual as well as group supervision, in which a group of trainees connects from the same site (R. J. Reese et al., 2009) or several trainees connect using multipoint video capabilities with a supervisor (Rousmaniere, Abbass, Frederickson, Henning, & Taubner, 2014). Group telesupervision has the advantage that the trainees learn from a supervisor and from each other. Telesupervision has also been used as a strategy to support and retain postdoctoral fellows and early professionals who are practicing in rural and remote areas, ranging from rural Nebraska to international venues such as Canada and Norway (Rousmaniere, Abbass, & Frederickson, 2014).

Real-time supervision with VC also offers exciting new training opportunities; the approach has been used with a handful of settings to date. With this model, the supervisor watches a live psychotherapy session over VC and gives feedback in real time. Feedback may be provided directly through audible prompts or through more sophisticated approaches such as the "bug in the ear" Bluetooth microphone that allows the supervisor to unobtrusively coach the trainee in a live session with a client/patient. The immediate feedback at crucial psychotherapy choice points offers a number of experiential learning advantages and permits state-dependent learning. Kobak, Craske, Rose, and Wolitsky-Taylor (2013) described role-play simulations of client interactions over VC, with the trainee role-playing the therapist role and the trainer role-playing an anxious client.

Another innovative telesupervision approach is the "virtual bedside teaching model" (Szeftel et al., 2011). In this model, the treatment room is equipped with technology for VC, sometimes even televideo robots that are capable of moving about, to observe the live interaction between a behavioral health provider/team and a client/family. Before beginning, the client/family consents to being observed by trainees. The approach has advantages as a group of trainees may observe without interfering with patient care, which is not feasible within traditional small clinic spaces. In a distant room, the supervisor uses the "live" interaction as a case-based springboard for discussion among the group. The distant room may be in the same location as the behavioral health sessions (i.e., the same building or campus) or it may at a different location. The use of the "mute" function allows the individuals in each room to "step out" of the virtual clinic mode and attend to their separate functions without completely disengaging from each other or the experience. This approach has been described with both psychiatric trainees (Szeftel et al., 2011) and trainees in child development clinics. In some cases, the trainee group may ask questions of the therapist in session to better understand the therapeutic approach.

In addition to VC, the range of telehealth technologies may be used for supervision, including telephone and e-mail supervision, supervision websites (Rousmaniere, Abbass, & Frederickson, 2014; Rousmaniere, Abbass, Frederickson, Henning, & Taubner, 2014), and even instant messenger services as demonstrated with peer-to-peer psychiatry learning in developing countries (Keynejad et al., 2013). New technology-supported consultation models are emerging to meet health care needs in underserved areas. The University of New Mexico pioneered one such model, Project ECHO (Extension of Healthcare Outcomes), with the goal of "demonopolizing knowledge" (Arora et al., 2014) and building capacity in rural primary care practices and other settings to deliver the same quality of care as care received at the academic health center (see http://echo.unm.edu/). The approach uses weekly group VC sessions with brief didactics followed by deidentified case presentations by the learners. Attendees therefore learn from the expert team and from each other and earn continuing education credit. On the basis of promising results that have demonstrated comparable, and in some cases better, outcomes than traditional services (Arora et al., 2011), the approach is growing nationally and internationally. The approach has expanded to dozens of complex and chronic conditions, including behavioral topics such as addiction, pain management, palliative care, attention-deficit/hyperactivity disorder, dementia, and others.

TELESUPERVISION PROCESS

To increase supervisor and trainee comfort, it is important to plan for the supervisory experience and mutually agree on key supervisory elements. Such agreement will help create the supportive, trusting environment in which the trainee feels comfortable openly sharing thoughts, ideas, experiences, and feelings with the supervisor. As in on-site supervision, this is crucial to advance trainee skills and, ultimately, provide high-quality patient care. Ongoing assessment of the supervisory experience from the perspectives of the supervisor and trainee(s) is strongly encouraged to continuously improve supervision when using technology. Short "process" comments about the supervision experience are therefore suggested.

In addition, telesupervision usually involves the transmission of patient protected health information and thus may fall under the Health Insurance Portability and Accountability Act (HIPAA). Therefore, the same level of care described in Chapter 2 of this volume concerning the transmission of clinical encounters should be undertaken for telesupervision encounters, documents, recordings, and technologies. Similarly, informed consent requirements also need to be followed (see Chapter 3).

As with on-site sessions, the supervisor needs to be skilled in assessing the individual and group personalities as well as goals that may influence the training experience. Strategies to maximize communication also need to be used to overcome potential challenges in fully observing nonverbal cues over VC. For example, it may be necessary to periodically pause and ask the trainee if he or she has questions given the potential delay in real-time VC connection or any other technical issues that may occur. Asking the trainee for feedback about the telesupervision process is also recommended.

Traditional, on-site supervisory strategies may be used in tandem with VC, including assigning readings, giving case presentations, jointly viewing videos, and sharing information through the multimedia capabilities of VC or through encrypted file sharing.

Telesupervision requires establishing the expectations of the trainee(s) and supervisor, ideally with a written understanding of expectations, responsibilities, and obligations over time. Key telesupervision questions include the following:

- Does the telesupervision approach meet the *trainee's need*, and are both the trainee and supervision engaged in telesupervision success?
- Does the supervisor have *cultural and linguistic competence* to meet the trainee's needs and the populations served by the trainee? If not, how can this deficiency be redressed?

- What *strengths and weaknesses* does the trainee bring to the supervisory relationship, including technology-specific areas? Does the supervisor feel inferior to the supervisee with respect to managing technology? Has this issue been adequately resolved?
- Which *technology* will meet this need? Is that technology secure and reliable? What are the backup plans if the technology does not work? Which technology support is needed, if any? Who will provide that tech support? What are their qualifications? Have they signed a technology security agreement, such as a Business Associate's Agreement if in the United States?
- What are the professional and local *regulatory requirements* for supervision provided through the use of technology? Are there limits on the number of hours that telesupervision can count toward licensure, continuing education credits, etc.? What counts as "supervision?" If there are technical difficulties for the first half of the supervisory session, what time will be counted as time spent in clinical supervision?
- What jurisdiction has *legal accountability* when supervision or training is conducted across state lines or international borders? Some states and provinces require that supervisees be licensed in the state of service delivered by the supervisee (Maheu, Pulier, Wilhelm, McMenamin, & Brown-Connolly, 2004; Rousmaniere, Abbass, & Frederickson, 2014; Rousmaniere, Abbass, Frederickson, Henning, & Taubner, 2014). Are other supervisors involved? If yes, where are all parties located geographically? Do other state or international laws apply?
- Do all professionals involved have *liability insurance* policies covering telesupervision?
- Will the supervisory *format* be group supervision or 1:1 supervision, or a combination?
- Will *all supervision be over technology, or will sessions be mixed* between on-site and VC supervision? For example, is e-mail or texting acceptable? If yes, which systems have been approved? Which types of communications are approved?
- What is the *frequency* of the supervision sessions and how are they scheduled? How are cancellations handled? What is the scheduling and

emergency contact information? What are the expectations around contacting each other in between sessions?

- What are the *documentation* and record-keeping requirements? Are there special considerations with electronic health record(s) in terms of trainee notes? If e-mails and text messages are being transmitted, where are they being documented?
- Will the trainee use *audio or video recording* of client/patient sessions as part of supervision? If recorded, how will recordings be stored securely? If in the United States, is the recorded file being scored in a HIPAA-secured environment, such as a cloud storage service that gives a Business Associate Agreement? Is the trainee privately recording any part of the exchange? Has recording been discussed?
- How will the supervisor and trainee *evaluate the supervisory sessions* and provide feedback? Are any related documents being exchanged in unencrypted e-mail?
- How will the supervisor complete *formal evaluation* about clinical progress, including meeting training program requirements?
- Is there a *financial relationship* between the trainee and supervisor?
- What are the expectations for *confidentiality* during the telesupervision sessions and any reasonably anticipated limits to confidentiality?
- What are the *legal requirements*, such as mandatory reporting requirements?
- How will the *termination* of the supervisory relationship be managed?

On the basis of these considerations, the supervisor and the trainee are encouraged to tailor an individualized telesupervision plan to meet the learning needs. This plan is revisited over time as the trainee advances in skills, with consideration to supervisory evaluation information and challenges related to changing technologies to further refine the supervision plan.

Supervisors must stay alert for cultural cues or miscommunications related to relevant local norms, laws, and regulations, noting verbal and nonverbal communication differences across cultures as well as language proficiency (see Chapter 6). For example, Rousmaniere, Abbass, Frederickson, Henning, and Taubner (2014) described supervision between American supervisors and Chinese trainees, including the culture's differences regarding in-group versus individual focus and pace of life. They reference a "triad model" in which the trainee has both an on-site and a VC supervisor. Inviting local supervisors to join the training experience may help acculturate the supervisee to rural or other local cultural norms (Wood, Miller, & Hargrove, 2005). As in the in-office setting, it is important to consider how the supervisor is a role model for the supervisee, including modeling best ethical practices as well as self-care and psychological wellness (Barnett & Molzon, 2014).

TRAINING AND COMPETENCE IN TELEPRACTICE

Because of the newness of the telepractice field, telepractice training approaches have evolved from the efforts of creative clinicians who have sought innovative solutions to better serve their patients. Thus, training has tended to be in the field, rather than in graduate school or other more formalized educational settings. As use of the Internet became more mainstream in the 1990s, clinicians often began the adoption of various Internet-mediated technologies without supervision or a comprehensive understanding of legal and ethical requirements (Maheu & Gordon, 2000). Lessons learned from these early experiences inform current training in telepractice and speak to the need to seek initial and ongoing training, supervision, and peer support when adopting new technologies (Barnett & Molzon, 2014; Callan, Maheu, & Bucky, in press).

The supervisor supports the trainee in delivering the highest quality care using technologies, minimizing harm and maximizing benefit. For some trainees, supervision may also encompass practice management/business development skills. Thus, supervisors need both a high level of competence in the theory and practice of telepractice, as well as in effective supervision. Telepractice training and supervision focus on developing and maintaining telemental health (TMH) competencies.

As in all areas of practice, TMH professional competence falls along a continuum; one is neither fully competent nor totally incompetent. The need for well-articulated competencies in training was identified by the Institute of Medicine (2001) in an effort to close the gap between training and improve initial and ongoing professional education. Progress has been made in overall behavioral health competencies, with examples such as the Health Service Psychology Education Collaborative (see http://www.ccptp.org/assets/docs/ccptp_presentation_the_health_service_psychology_education_collaborative_blueprint_belar_02-2013.pdf). These overall efforts provide a foundation for competencies specific to telepractice and the associated training to meet these competencies in post- and prelicensure training.

Postlicensure Training

Acquiring the new telepractice competencies can be daunting given the rapid pace of both technology change and overall changes in health care. New trainees have often "caught the technology bug" and are eager to learn about telepractice and initiate services. Supervisors assist trainees in considering all aspects of telepractice and the competencies associated with thoughtful, cautious, and responsible telepractice (Maheu, 2003). They also assist in setting realistic goals for building these telepractice skills over time to provide the highest quality care.

One of the earliest telepractice competency models is the online clinical practice management model published by Maheu (2003; Maheu et al., 2004). This important road map outlines seven competency areas: (a) training, (b) referral practices, (c) client education, (d) legal issues, (e) intake and assessment, (f) direct care, and (g) reimbursement procedures. Similarly, the Ohio Psychological Association (2013) encouraged practitioners and their supervisors embarking on telepractice to conduct a self-assessment of

- knowledge and skills of technology approaches;
- knowledge and skills of clinical telepractice;
- knowledge and skills for establishing, maintaining, and terminating the telepractitioner and client relationship;
- supervisor and supervisee knowledge and skills of technology approaches;
- knowledge and skills for establishing, maintaining, and terminating supervisor and supervisee relationship; and
- ongoing professional development requirements and continuing education to maintain current knowledge and skill competencies in telepractice.

These types of self-assessment can assist the trainee and supervisor to identify training gaps; develop a realistic plan that sets goals that address these gaps; implement the training plan; and, after an agreed-on time period, assess progress toward the goal. It is not uncommon that a trainee will ultimately become a supervisor for new telepractice trainees.

Prelicensure Training

For students in training, supervised TMH experiences are the exception rather than the rule. Very few predoctoral and internship programs have TMH rotations, with the exception of the Veterans Affairs and a handful of rural-focused programs (Duncan, Nelson, et al., 2013). In psychology, recent progress has been made as TMH-related experiences now count toward clinical hours on the Association of Psychology Postdoctoral and Internship Centers application (see http://www.appic.org). Dunstan and Tooth (2012) described training value related to clinical psychology trainees providing VC services to patients with depression and anxiety. Colbow (2013) also presented strategies to integrate TMH into psychologist training that can readily be applied across behavioral and mental health professions.

At the most basic level, prelicensure trainees may be in the same room observing an established telepractitioner as he or she videoconferences with diverse clients across the range of diagnoses and geographies, without ever leaving his or her desk. Trainees may first observe the telepractitioner and then progress to providing technology-based services themselves.

In contrast to on-site clinic rooms, multiple trainees may observe the telepractice session "in the background," without crowding the client and potentially impacting clinical care. The trainee and supervisor always gain the client's permission for trainees (or supervisors) to observe unobtrusively in the background or off screen. The telepractice supervisor may support trainees with readings such as national guidelines (APA, 2013a; Grady et al., 2011; Turvey et al., 2013), review articles (Gros et al., 2013; Slone, Reese, & McClellan, 2012), or more intensive textbooks (Maheu et al., 2004; Myers & Turvey, 2012). "Mock" videos of telepractice sessions help trainees gain a better understanding of similarities and differences between telepractice and on-site practice. Supervisors often emphasize that telepractice is not "half" service but approximates all key elements of best ethical care on-site.

Nelson, Bui, and Sharp (2011) described this approach in which a range of trainees (e.g., psychology, social work, psychiatry, and pediatrics trainees) observed the TeleHelp clinic, an interdisciplinary telemedicine clinic treating youth depression. The team emphasized four key trainee competencies:

- proficiency with evidence-based assessment and treatment of youth depression;
- cultural competence across ethnicity, language, socioeconomic, and other individual characteristics (e.g., medical status, psychiatric stability, physical/cognitive disability, and personal preferences; APA, 2013a; see also Chapter 9, this volume), as well as overall literacy and health literacy awareness;
- technology competencies, in this case proficiency with room-based videoconferencing; and
- communication competencies in working with the interdisciplinary team, as well as with the system of care and communities.

TELEPRACTICE TRAINING RESOURCES

A common model for behavioral health professionals who have never participated in telepractice is to seek early training and shadowing opportunities with established TMH practitioners in their local settings. Individuals seeking additional intensive training may seek out on-site opportunities in telemedicine, covering a range of telepractice topics that mirror TMH topics within this book. When there are few or no TMH providers in the trainee's community, it may also be valuable to observe experienced telepractitioners in other specialties.

Clinical providers may also seek on-site and online training opportunities specific to evidence-based best practices in behavioral health across technologies. For less intense opportunities, individuals may pursue training opportunities through technology-related groups within their broader professional organization (e.g., technology special interest group of the Society of Behavioral Medicine); workshops featuring TMH leaders at annual state, provincial, or national conventions; or behavioral-health groups within broader telehealth or technology-focused groups (e.g., the TMH special interest group through the American Telemedicine Association or the Coalition for Technology in Behavioral Science). Such groups often make available networking and mentoring opportunities. Online communities of like-minded professionals are also available through TMH training institutes and a variety of social media websites.

Innovative publications are also beginning to surface to help clinicians find more information about how to get involved with technology. Maheu, Drude, and Wright (2015) wrote a "field guide" to allow behavioral professionals to sample synopses of career paths as described by approximately 30 professionals who have bridged their medical or graduate training in behavioral care to involvement with technology. The field guide bears witness to the range of experiences that can inspire and nurture behavioral professionals seeking a rich and personally rewarding path to working in behavioral care by using 21st-century tools.

In the United States, the federally funded Telehealth Resource Centers (TRCs; http://www.telehealthresourcecenter.org/) provide up-to-date resources related to general telehealth practices, as well as linkages to meet the trainee needs. The TRCs and other organizations provide webinars that can serve as introductory samples of training for specific topic areas. The *Telemental Health Guide* (http://www.tmhguide.org/) also provides practical online information about key training topics, as well as on-demand library searches.

Fortunately, there is increasing guidance about effective strategies associated with developing and maintaining the comprehensive competencies associated with telepractice. Supervision and consultation with VC offers exciting opportunities to extend support to health care providers and trainees, wherever they may be. Just as in clinical practice, careful attention must be taken to translate supervisory and training practices to the telehealth setting.

9

Ethical Telepractice With Diverse Populations

Technology makes it possible to provide telemental health (TMH) services in real time with clients across the city, the state, the country, or even the world. Thus, telepractice has the potential to improve access for underserved and vulnerable populations and, ultimately, to address health disparities. With this expanded reach, it has become even more important that telepractitioners carefully question and assess their competence with diverse populations. Following ethical best practices, clinicians consider the populations' unique needs related to both the behavioral health and the technology aspects of telepractice.

The American Psychological Association (APA, 2010a) *Ethical Principles of Psychologists and Code of Conduct* emphasizes close attention to the needs of diverse populations across training, practice, and research. Under Principle E: Respect for People's Rights and Dignity, it reminds

http://dx.doi.org/10.1037/14938-010
A Practitioner's Guide to Telemental Health: How to Conduct Legal, Ethical, and Evidence-Based Telepractice, by D. D. Luxton, E.-L. Nelson, and M. M. Maheu

clinicians to "be aware of and respect cultural, individual, and role differences, including those based on age, gender, gender identity, race, ethnicity, culture, national origin, religion, sexual orientation, disability, language, and socioeconomic status and consider these factors" (p. 4). Very similar guidance is provided through the codes of ethics of the National Association of Social Workers (2008) and the American Counseling Association (2014). Similarly, the American Psychiatric Association reflects a number of position statements related to diversity (see http://www.psychiatry.org), and the American Academy of Child and Adolescent Psychiatry's Practice Parameter sets forth principles of cultural competence as professionals work with children, adolescents, and their families (http://www.jaacap.com/article/S0890-8567(13)00479-6/pdf).

Overall, *cultural humility* (Hook, Davis, Owen, Worthington, & Utsey, 2013) is strongly encouraged, recognizing the lifelong, process-oriented approach to striving toward competency with the vulnerable groups served through technology. More specifically, the APA's *Guidelines for Providers of Psychological Services to Ethnic, Linguistic, and Culturally Diverse Populations* (APA Task Force, 1990) may be readily applied to telepractice. As noted by the APA Presidential Task Force (2013), cultural competence involves three broad dimensions: therapists' cultural knowledge, therapists' attitudes and beliefs toward culturally different clients and self-understanding, and therapists' skills and use of culturally appropriate interventions (see also APA Presidential Task Force, 2012).

Clinicians also strive to be aware of how their own cultural background/experiences, attitudes, values, and biases influence telepractice. As in traditional in-office settings, telepractitioners obtain the training, experience, consultation, or supervision necessary to ensure the competence of their services, or they make appropriate referrals (APA, 2002; Falender, Shafranske, & Falicov, 2014; see also Chapter 8, this volume). Teleproviders must be particularly mindful of these factors when working with immigrant-origin populations (APA Presidential Task Force, 2013).

With this ethical focus in mind, this chapter provides an overview of cultural considerations in telepractice. The process of initiating and sustaining services is described, as well as communication and relationship factors when working with patients across geographies (rural, suburban, and urban) and in homebound settings. Finally, strategies to support culturally aware telepractitioner competencies when working with diverse populations are summarized.

TIPS FOR INITIATING TELEPRACTICE

Telepractitioners pay close attention to the cultural aspects of the professional relationship. Culture is defined by the *Diagnostic and Statistical Manual of Mental Disorders* (fifth ed.; American Psychiatric Association, 2013) as "systems of knowledge, concepts, rules and practices that are learned and transmitted across generations. Culture includes language, religion and spirituality, family structure, life-cycles stages, ceremonial rituals, and customs, as well as moral and legal systems" (p. 749). Clients/patients in today's world are influenced by multiple cultures, making it crucial not to overgeneralize cultural information or stereotype groups. In telepractice, a thorough cultural formulation of the client/patient is essential, including cultural identity of the individual, cultural conceptualizations of distress, psychosocial stressors and resilience, and cultural features of the client–therapist relationship. Other key telepractice elements include assessment of the impact of culture on the client/patient's (a) overall comfort/socialization with the behavioral health system; (b) comfort and familiarity with the technology; (c) communication, rapport, and trust; and (d) perceptions of confidentiality.

Stigma

In some communities, there is greater stigma associated with behavioral and mental health for a variety of reasons. For example, some rural clients/patients may have an increased perception of confidentiality with therapists outside their own communities, thereby avoiding the dual relationships inherent in small, close-knit communities (Smalley, Warren, & Rainer, 2012). Seeking treatment for some health conditions may be perceived as stigmatizing within particular communities (e.g., developing countries, rural areas, and other settings). According to Earnshaw, Bogart, Dovidio, and Williams (2013), because of potential mistrust of the behavioral health system, particularly among individuals at risk for multiple stigmas (e.g., HIV positive, racial/ethnic, substance abuse), care should be taken to discuss confidentiality and its limits within the client's unique situation (see Chapter 3). Telepractice may be a treatment delivery solution for individuals who are hesitant to seek treatment for behavioral health concerns, such as the lesbian, gay, bisexual, transgender, queer and intersex (LGBTQI) community. For example, gender identity has been linked with increased smoking prevalence in rural gender minorities, who often get no specialized care for their underlying distress or smoking (Bennet, McElroy, Johnson, Munk, & Everett, 2015). Telehealth, then, offers many other types of people an effective way to receive highly specialized care in a nonstigmatizing manner. Another example is genetic counseling, which is virtually nonexistent in rural and remote areas (Hilgart, Hayward, Coles, & Iredale, 2012).

Geographical Settings

Telepractice offers the clinician the advantage of being able to see clients/patients from very different locations all in the same day via VC, potentially seeing a child at a rural primary care clinic, followed by a child at an urban middle school, and then a family in a frontier clinic. However, such a geographically mobile telepractitioner must be aware of and compensate for the challenges of such a practice by adjusting to local norms and resources associated with each of the geographic areas visited. Each geographical setting (e.g., urban, suburban, and rural) comprises diverse populations. Assumptions should therefore be avoided (Smalley, Warren, & Rainer, 2012); in lay terms: If you've seen one rural community then you've seen one rural community.

Seeking community input from community leaders, religious leaders, other respected elders, as well as schools and other organized groups is important with regard to understanding the economic climate (e.g., downturns resulting from droughts or factory closings), values (e.g., role of the faith community), and needs of vulnerable populations (e.g., migrant workers). Firearms are more accepted in some rural communities, and telepractitioners need to talk with staff and clients/patients about safety and risk management (Grady et al., 2011). Urban culture should also be considered when providing telepractice services. For example, there is increased risk of community violence in some urban neighborhoods served by urban telemedicine programs. It is essential that the teleprovider both understand the behavioral health needs associated with this risk (e.g., posttrauma reactions, grief) as well as be aware of community resources to support patients, their families, and their neighbors. Telepractice may be the option of choice for treatment because of feelings of disenfranchisement and distrust of the traditional medical system, even when the providers and clients/patients are located nearby.

Scheduling can be a challenge because clients/patients in underserved areas may hold several jobs with little control of their free time and be caring for their immediate and extended family as well as friends, dealing with their own illnesses, having difficulty securing consistent transportation, and experiencing other barriers. Unstable housing may also be a challenge, with families changing locations and schools before treatment is complete. With school-based TMH, the presenter is often a trusted school nurse who helps not only with the technology, but also with socializing the client/patient and family to behavioral health services and helping to follow up with recommendations (Spaulding, Cain, & Sonnenschein, 2011). Although telepractice has not been widely used with suburban populations, the need may increase given gaps in care associated with the growing numbers of people living with poverty in the suburbs (Kneebone & Berube, 2014).

Technical Considerations

The VC technology itself offers both benefits and challenges, depending on the individual client/patient. For example, some clients with hearing impairment may benefit because they are able to zoom in on the therapist's face to better read lips and can also turn up the volume. On the other hand, clients/patients with hearing impairment or cognitive impairment may find the slight delay in audio a challenge to communication.

When delivering services to older adults in home or residential settings, the interface between the client/patient and technology should be carefully considered, including the ease of use and the fit with the elders' mobility, dexterity, sight, and hearing. Given that broadband Internet access greatly facilitates the effective use of VC, it is wise to ask questions about any client/patient's technical capacity before making assumptions about age or ethnicity. For example, a 2014 Pew Research Center report (Smith, 2014b) showed that not all older people are the same when it comes to broadband. Older adult broadband use varied by age, household income, and education attainment. Similarly, broadband use varied by ethnicity, with African Americans trailing behind Whites in overall Internet use, home broadband access, and to a lesser degree mobile platforms (Smith, 2014a) and with Hispanics as a whole having high adoption rates with mobile technologies (Lopez, Gonzalez-Barrera, & Patten, 2013).

Feedback across the consumers, caregivers, telepractitioner, and community assists in developing culturally sensitive protocols, as well as periodically revising the protocols on the basis of multi-informant input (Brooks et al., 2013). The majority of published psychotherapy research in telepractice reports cognitive behavioral strategies, which may translate particularly well to the telepractice setting because of the practical, skills-focused approaches (Nelson & Duncan, 2015). It is important to note, however, that there are no traditional theoretical orientations, strategies, or approaches that have been excluded from telepractice with any one population.

Telepractice Environment

Telepractitioners strive to create a welcoming environment at both the clinician and the client/patient site. In supervised settings, the TMH space should be fully accessible to the population served, including wheelchair accessibility. When working with children, developmentally appropriate materials should be available (e.g., toys, drawing materials) and extraneous distractions should be removed (Cain, Nelson, & Myers, 2015). If providing services to children with behavioral disorders that put them at risk for destructive outbursts, the room at the distant site should be free of things that may be destroyed, and the distant personnel should be trained ahead of time regarding support expectations should the client have an outburst (Duncan, Velasquez, & Nelson, 2014).

Because some populations may have had no or very limited access to behavioral and mental health services, individuals may present with a higher level of acuity and comorbidity because of delays to treatment. These access problems may impact the telepractitioner's planning for length and frequency of sessions. Telepractitioners working with populations with limited resources may feel internal and external pressures to serve as many clients/patients as possible. Nonetheless, telepractitioners must continually assess their scope of practice and seek additional training, supervision, or consultation (see Chapter 8) when warranted.

Informed Consent

When obtaining informed consent to treatment, pay close attention to the client/patient's language preferences, general literacy needs, and health literacy needs (see also Chapter 3). The needs of the specific population should be considered. For example, when serving populations with cognitive impairment, telepractitioners should pay close attention to the client/patient's understanding and ability to give consent. Moreover, acculturation should be considered when obtaining consent, especially when providing services to immigrant and refugee populations. As in on-site clinical settings, special caution should be taken with consenting vulnerable populations such as children in foster care as well as inmates/prisoners (Batastini, McDonald, & Morgan, 2012). In addition, when providing telepractice services in a group setting, group members should be socialized to confidentiality expectations around the information shared with each other. It is also important to be mindful of how some groups may be accepting of telepractice as long as it is not recorded.

Using Interpreters and Community Health Workers

The client/patient's preferred language should be considered when delivering VC services. Best practices in medical interpreting are encouraged (Brooks et al., 2013), including seeking a trained interpreter rather than relying on family members for a pediatric patient. Additionally, there are several companies that offer interpreting services via VC, across languages including sign language. Several TMH research reports have noted client preference for bilingual therapists from the same cultural background (Chong & Moreno, 2012; Ye et al., 2012), although this may not be feasible. Other innovative solutions include using asynchronous telepsychiatry consults with Spanish speaking clients (Yellowlees et al., 2013).

A number of TMH programs use community health workers (CHW), also known as community health advocates, lay health educators, community health representatives, *promotores de salud/promotoras*, and other terms. They serve as patient-friendly connectors between health care consumers and the health care system. Because CHWs live in the communities they serve, they can advance telepractice by supporting the client/patient in the encounter and informing the telepractitioner about local cultural norms and current events that impact the community. For example, with American Indian Veterans, a tribal/telehealth outreach worker supports the client and facilitates establishing trust and rapport (Brooks et al., 2013).

Last, partnerships with advocates and policy makers looking toward telepractice to address health disparities may be considered. For example, the National Organization of Black Elected Legislative Women (http://www.nobel-women.org) spearheads policy change to extend telepractice to underserved women and children.

OPTIMIZING COMMUNICATION AND THERAPEUTIC RELATIONSHIPS

In terms of relationship building and communication, telepractice has varying impact across diverse populations. As in the traditional clinic setting, the clinician should also take variability within the group into consideration and assess individual client/patient preferences. Some clients/patients may find the additional control and anonymity afforded by the telepractice setting appealing, as reported with veteran populations who have experienced trauma (Brooks et al., 2013), nursing home residents, or correctional facility populations (Maheu, Pulier, Wilhelm, McMenamin, & Brown-Connolly, 2004). Similarly, adolescents have been reported to quickly accommodate to the technology setting and often like the additional "personal space" offered by telepractice (Cain, Nelson, & Myers, 2015). It has been reported that Caucasian clients may find decreased direct eye contact a challenge. On the other hand, some Asian and Native American clients have been reported to prefer the decreased direct eye contact (Brooks et al., 2013; Shore, Savin, Novins, & Manson, 2006).

Across populations, it remains important for telepractitioners to carefully attend to both verbal and nonverbal communication clues. The telepractitioner should pay attention to norms of communication within the client/patient's culture. For instance, storytelling approaches may be common in some American Indian cultures, and additional time should be used to accommodate this preferred style (Brooks et al., 2013). As discussed in Chapter 6, telepractitioners may verbally "check in" with clients to ask about their experience of the technology. Good lighting is important to note facial expressions across ethnicities and emotional expressions such as crying.

Because telepractice allows clients/patients to be seen while remaining in their own communities, there are advantages to increased numbers of family members and related supporters participating in sessions. This family-focused approach has been noted as particularly appealing to some Hispanic clients (Santiago-Rivera, Arredondo, & Gallardo-Cooper, 2002). Telepractitioners should consider practicalities such as rooms large enough to accommodate extended families with many family members, as well as who will assist with managing those in the room and to ensure confidential communication when talking with the participants individually. Emerging technologies also offer advantages to allow family members to join the session by multiple-point VC. For example, adult children living in a distant state could join a palliative care social support meeting to support a parent who has provided consent for their participation.

TELEPRACTICE EXAMPLES WITH VULNERABLE POPULATIONS

It is important for TMH practitioners to be familiar with best practices when working with vulnerable populations. These populations include persons who have experienced traumas (e.g., war, sexual assault, accidents, violence), patients with certain types of health conditions, homebound patients, and others.

Traumatized Clients/Patients

Despite clinical advances in treating traumatized adults and children, very few individuals who have experienced trauma receive evidence-based care, often because of workforce shortages (U.S. Department of Health and Human Services, Substance Abuse and Mental Health Services Administration, 2013b). Telepractice helps bridge this gap and better serve vulnerable groups across varied types of trauma, as well as increase trauma intervention training opportunities. TMH research has shown much promise in helping traumatized populations. As Gros et al. (2013) summarized, cognitive behavioral therapy interventions delivered face-to-face and using VC were equally effective in improving overall functioning for veterans with posttraumatic stress disorder as well as in community populations. Innovative, patient-centered models are emerging with home-based services (Strachan et al., 2012) and collaborative care (Fortney et al., 2015). Telepractice has also been shown as beneficial for women veterans who have experienced sexual assault during their military service (Lutwak & Dill, 2013), as well as for women in the community who have experienced domestic violence (Hassija & Gray, 2011).

Limited TMH research has addressed telepractice and trauma in pediatric populations. Telepractice offers unique advantages around providing specialized expertise to evaluate child sexual abuse. In fact, rural hospitals using telemedicine for pediatric sexual abuse forensic examination consultations provided significantly higher quality evaluations, more complete examinations, and more accurate diagnoses than similar hospitals conducting examinations without telemedicine support and without access to pediatric specialists in these areas (Miyamoto et al., 2014).

Clients/Patients With Health Conditions

Telepractice also has great potential to connect behavioral providers specializing in health conditions. Children with obesity, feeding difficulties, cancer, diabetes, congenital heart disorder, epilepsy, cystic fibrosis, and other conditions have successfully received pediatric psychology services over VC (Nelson & Patton, in press). With adults, telepractice research has focused on medical aspects of HIV care with a wide variety of groups (Maheu et al., 2004), including veterans (Saifu et al., 2012), incarcerated individuals (Young et al., 2014), and individuals in their homes (León et al., 2011). Some studies have suggested that participants may find telehealth more private than health care at their on-site clinic because of reduced anxiety regarding encountering any members of their community or acquaintances (Saberi, Yuan, John, Sheon, & Johnson, 2013).

Homebound Patients and Caregivers

Another population that telepractitioners may serve is homebound patients with severe functional impairments, life-limiting conditions, and/or rehabilitation concerns (American Telemedicine Association, 2010). Given the variability of such patients, telepractice appropriateness should be determined on a case-by-case basis, with selections based on clinical judgment, client's informed choice, and professional standards of care.

Homebound clients and their families often experience high levels of isolation, fears about functional decline and death, and diminishing quality of life, as well as depression, concerns about caregivers, financial worries, and day-to-day stressors associated with challenging medical regimens. Home-based TMH may decrease risks associated with travel (e.g., infection control risks, discomfort) in critically ill populations, such as patients with amyotrophic lateral sclerosis (ALS; McClellan, Washington, Ruff, & Selkirk, 2013) and children on ventilators (Casavant, McManus, Parsons, Zurakowski, & Graham, 2014). TMH addresses challenges in driving associated with vision loss, seizures, cognitive difficulties, and other conditions. However, home-based services are not yet fully reimbursed through third-party payers.

When working with individuals who are homebound, the professional, patient, and caregivers review whether the intervention will focus on the patient, the caregiver, or both. They agree on the areas of focus, which may include behavioral medicine strategies associated with coping with the condition and adhering to the medical regimen; assistance with communication with the medical team; intervention related to psychiatric concerns, such as depression, couples or family therapy, palliative care support, support for caregivers, and other areas specific to the homebound patient's needs. The teleprovider may be a member of the patient's overall treatment team or may be external to this team; communication and care coordination across treatment providers should be discussed with the patient and caregiver as part of the informed consent process.

The telepractitioner may use creativity in considering the range of possible telepractice services that may support the mental health and well-being of the client/patient and their caregivers. For example, VC delivery of interventions ranging from tai chi (Tousignant et al., 2014) to resilience-focused psychoeducation (Nelson, Mulhern, Bush, & Groneman, 2011) may improve quality of life. Support groups using VC directly to the home may be cost-effective resources to support the homebound client and family (Kim et al., 2014). In addition, emerging technologies for behavioral health purposes such as instant messaging have been reported to be a good fit for patients experiencing cognitive impairment as a means to address memory deficits (Forducey, Glueckauf, Bergquist, Maheu, & Yutsis, 2012).

Telepractitioners and clients/patients should discuss expectations for availability, including whether the telepractitioners will be available only during scheduled times or are also available for consultation with emergent concerns. For example, telepractitioners serving hospice patients (Oliver et al., 2012) sometimes have extended availability in supporting the dying patient and their families. The telepractitioner and client also establish a plan should the client's health deteriorate during the session.

Finally, Chi and Demiris (2015) presented a comprehensive review of how telepractice may support caregivers. Across 65 studies with caregivers of adult and pediatric patients, six main categories of interventions were identified: education, consultation (including decision support), psychosocial/cognitive–behavioral therapy, social support, data collection and monitoring, and clinical care delivery. More than 95% of the studies reported significant improvements in the caregivers' outcomes and that caregivers were satisfied and comfortable with telehealth.

10

Conclusion

As we have discussed throughout this guidebook, telemental health (TMH) and other health technologies provide numerous advantages and benefits to both care providers and care seekers, including enhanced access to care, decreased travel and related costs, greater community support, reduced stigma, and convenience. Key drivers of TMH expansion include health care reform, a continued shift toward patient/family-centric health care delivery, cost savings, technological advancements, and decreased technology costs. This final chapter provides a review of these drivers and the rationale for behavioral health providers to not only embrace technology but also lead technological adoption as needed "behavior change" for other health care disciplines. We first describe expanded TMH settings and services, including primary care, home-based services, and stepped-care models that include the range of health technologies. We then address emerging technology options that advance TMH.

http://dx.doi.org/10.1037/14938-011
A Practitioner's Guide to Telemental Health: How to Conduct Legal, Ethical, and Evidence-Based Telepractice, by D. D. Luxton, E.-L. Nelson, and M. M. Maheu

EXPANDED TELEMENTAL HEALTH SETTINGS AND SERVICES

Increasing numbers of individual care providers, health-related institutions, and governments are recognizing the value of providing behavioral and mental health care via technology to decrease spiraling costs related to neglected behavioral health care. The need is compelling in the United States (U.S. Department of Health and Human Services, Substance Abuse and Mental Health Services Administration, 2013a). The majority of adults and children with behavioral health needs does not receive any services, let alone evidence-based assessment and treatment from trained mental health professionals (Merikangas et al., 2011).

In the United States, more people have health insurance, especially with the passage of the Patient Protection and Affordable Care Act in 2010, and behavioral health coverage has expanded with the Mental Health Parity and Addiction Equity Act of 2008. Reimbursements for telehealth services have also been expanded and can be expected to extend to more types of services. As of 2015, videoconferencing-based telehealth services can be reimbursed in all 50 states by Medicare and in 46 of states by Medicaid (http://cchpca.org/state-telehealth-laws-and-reimbursement-policies-report). In many of these states, some telehealth-based services are covered in parity with in-person care. Telehealth coverage is on the horizon for Accountable Care Organizations under the Centers for Medicaid and Medicare Services (American Telemedicine Association [ACA], 2014). Expansion of telehealth in the United States is also driving worldwide trends, which are expected to grow substantially over the next few years to increase access to quality care (IHS, 2014).

With health care reform, primary care practices are becoming increasingly important in behavioral health services, both because of the high prevalence of behavioral health concerns at office visits and because of the patient's trusted relationship with the primary care provider and treatment team. The ACA-mandated reforms in the structure, functioning, and financing of primary care that provide many opportunities for TMH (Myers & Lieberman, 2013). TMH may advance behaviorally oriented integrated care models in primary care by providing direct behavioral services and supporting teleconsultation with behavioral health specialists. TMH also helps underserved primary care settings, including Federally Qualified Health Centers and other community sites, by advancing patient-centered medical home (PCMH) goals and PCMH recognition/designation. Legislative reform worldwide can be expected to focus on the integration of a wide range of services, including behavioral services to medical patients.

As growing consumer demand facilitates telehealth adoption, there are an increasing number of opportunities to use TMH to connect multiple settings and systems to advance care coordination. For instance, it is technologically feasible to connect the patient, family, behavioral health specialists, primary care provider, and school representatives at the same time for the assessment and treatment of child behavioral concerns to set common goals and problem solve (Duncan, Velasquez, & Nelson, 2014; Nelson & Patton, in press).

In addition to traditional TMH services, behavioral medicine and health psychology services over telehealth are becoming increasingly important. CMS and other insurers look toward creative solutions to meet the needs of "super utilizers" of hospitals and emergency department services, the majority of whom have co-occurring behavioral health concerns in addition to multiple chronic illnesses. TMH services have the potential to enhance care coordination and adherence, prevent the need for hospital stays, lead to considerable cost savings, and improve the quality of life for these clients/patients and their caregivers (Chakravarty, Cantor, Walkup, & Tong, 2014; Luxton, 2013).

TMH services also go hand-in-hand with new distance educational models aimed at increasing primary care capacity to care for complex, chronic illnesses. For example, Project ECHO (Extension of Community Healthcare Outcomes; see http://echo.unm.edu/) uses telehealth technologies and case-based learning with an interprofessional teams to build rural and underserved practice capacity to deliver the same, or better, quality of care as received at academic institutions (Arora et al., 2014). TMH also has growing potential to advance prevention and public health initiatives as communities shift to a "culture of health" (see http://www.rwjf.org/en/about-rwjf/annual-reports/presidents-message-2014.html). This includes

TMH services focused on weight management, smoking cessation, and stress management. Finally, there is potential to expand use and training/support of community health workers and to increase mental health supports for diverse populations (Shore et al., 2012).

Home-based TMH is yet another burgeoning area that offers many advantages to support patients and their families in a convenient, client-friendly environment. It allows the telepractitioner a "window into the home" to conduct in vivo treatment, including supporting family members. Research and consensus building has led to effective strategies to deliver high quality, safe service right to the client/patient's home. This validated approach requires properly educating the clinicians as well as the recipient(s) of care (Luxton, O'Brien, McCann, & Mishkind, 2012; Maheu, Pulier, Wilhelm, McMenamin, & Brown-Connolly, 2004). Although home-based TMH services are not generally reimbursed through public and private insurers, there are many advocacy initiatives supporting this goal. Moreover, CPT (Current Procedural Terminology) billing code changes are preparing the way for such reimbursement by including codes for consultation with family members "with and without" direct patient involvement.

Clinical guidelines written by different professional groups frequently recommend that services for depression, anxiety, and other behavioral health conditions be structured around a stepped care model. In these models, clients/patients receive treatment at increasing "steps" or levels of treatment intensity (i.e., the amount and type), increasing at each step if they continue to experience distress at previous steps (Bower & Gilbody, 2005; L'Abate, 2013; Richards et al., 2012). Stepped care includes a continuum of guided self-help/self-management, progressing to traditional behavioral health options such as therapy. In addition, treatment progress is closely monitored to inform stepped care decision making.

TMH advances the stepped care model in two ways. First, technology, such as mHealth apps, extends options for close and more immediate monitoring of client/patient symptoms, informing when the next step of care is needed. Second, the vast array of asynchronous and synchronous technologies, such as behavioral health web-based services and videoconferencing (VC), offers evidence-supported behavioral options across self-care and treatment needs. For example, a client/patient with significant stress and warning signs of depression may first use a stress management app (Luxton, Hansen, & Stanfill, 2014) and a self-guided online depression intervention. If the individual's symptoms persist or worsen, he or she progresses to the next level of a technology-supported care, and synchronous VC services with health care providers may be added for ongoing therapy or crisis management.

EXPANDED TELEMENTAL HEALTH TECHNOLOGY OPTIONS

The accessibility of inexpensive technologies such as webcams, Internet-based VC software, and mobile device apps greatly enhances a professional's capabilities to provide quality services. With the exception of underserved and very remote areas, most communities now have affordable and readily available high-speed connectivity options. Although discouraged for clinical purposes because of security and related considerations (see Chapter 3, this volume), Skype and FaceTime's popularity for social purposes has increased consumer understanding and comfort with VC. This familiarity with VC has encouraged the adoption of more health care appropriate VC platforms.

A variety of other new health technologies are on the horizon. This includes innovations such as virtual reality, augmented reality, intelligent wearable devices, and artificial intelligence applications used for clinical care (Luxton, 2015). Virtual artificial intelligent agents, for example, make use of virtual reality and artificial intelligence techniques including machine learning and natural language processing (Luxton, 2014a, 2015). This enables intelligent virtual simulation of human practitioners that can converse with the client/patient in real time. These systems have the potential to be accessed via the Internet 24/7 and can augment what psychologists and other mental health professional do by providing coaching, training, and other therapeutic functions (Luxton, 2014a, 2014b, 2015). In another example, robots with synchronous video capabilities can travel from hospital room to hospital room and allow care providers to speak with patients from remote locations through the onboard video system. This has the potential to assist a telepsychiatrist staffing an inpatient setting to interact with patients in crisis. There is also potential for hospitalized and homebound children with critically ill conditions to videoconference with their classrooms and friends using robots. These types of technological developments, although not widely adopted at present, promise to bring new capabilities to enhance behavioral health care.

SUMMARY

As does traditional on-site practice, TMH rests on behavioral and mental health practitioners' dedication to providing the highest quality ethical and legal services to their clients/patients. Although this guidebook advocates the adoption of video-based technologies for behavioral and mental health care, it also cautions against jumping too quickly into unknown waters. TMH is advanced by caring practitioners who respond with creativity and innovation to clients/patients in need and their families. Such professional use of technology is based in comprehensive graduate education or postgraduate professional training, supervision, and consultation. Lifelong learning and peer-to-peer support are encouraged as behavioral health professionals initiate and sustain telepractice. TMH competency rests on keeping up-to-date with the scientific evidence base (Cain, Nelson, & Myers, 2015; Hilty et al., 2013; Shore et al., 2014), as well as ongoing collegial discussion with informed leaders in the clinical, ethical, and legal telehealth arenas of relevance.

The requirements for ensuring safe, competent, and ethical TMH are not to be feared. Practitioners who adhere to the latest practice guidelines, gain specialized training for TMH, and apply the knowledge and skills they already have as behavioral health professionals can be confident that they are providing a rewarding, safe, reliable, and quality care option. TMH is a powerful way to help behavioral and mental health professionals decrease patient suffering by expanding best practices in health prevention, assessment, treatment, maintenance/support, and consultation.

References

American Counseling Association. (2014). *ACA code of ethics.* Retrieved from http://www.counseling.org/Resources/aca-code-of-ethics.pdf

American Psychiatric Association. (2013). *Diagnostic and statistical manual of mental disorders* (5th ed.). Washington, DC: Author.

American Psychological Association. (2002). Ethical principles of psychologists and code of conduct. *American Psychologist, 57*, 1060–1073. Retrieved from http://www.apa.org/ethics/code/

American Psychological Association. (2010a). *Ethical principles of psychologists and code of conduct (2002, Amended June 1, 2010).* Retrieved from http://www.apa.org/ethics/code/index.aspx

American Psychological Association. (2010b). Telepsychology is on the rise. *Monitor on Psychology, 41*(3), 11.

American Psychological Association. (2013a). *Guidelines for the practice of telepsychology.* Retrieved from http://www.apapracticecentral.org/ce/guidelines/telepsychology-guidelines.pdf

American Psychological Association. (2013b). *Telepsychology 50-state review.* Retrieved from http://www.apapracticecentral.org/advocacy/state/telehealth-slides.pdf

American Psychological Association. (2014). Are psychologists in the states that have the most mental illness? *Monitor on Psychology, 45*(10), 13. Retrieved from http://www.apa.org/monitor/2014/11/datapoint.aspx

American Psychological Association Presidential Task Force on Immigration. (2013). *Working with immigrant-origin clients: An update for mental health professionals.* Washington, DC: Author. Retrieved from http://www.apa.org/topics/immigration/immigration-report-professionals.pdf

American Psychological Association Presidential Task Force on Preventing Discrimination and Promoting Diversity. (2012). *Dual pathways to a better America: Preventing discrimination and promoting diversity.* Washington, DC: Author. http://www.apa.org/pubs/info/reports/promoting-diversity.aspx

American Psychological Association Task Force on the Delivery of Services to Ethnic and Minority Populations. (1990). *Guidelines for providers of psychological services to ethnic, linguistic, and culturally diverse populations.* Washington, DC: Author. Retrieved from http://www.apa.org/pi/oema/resources/policy/provider-guidelines.aspx

American Telemedicine Association. (2009). *Practice guidelines for videoconferencing-based telemental health.* Retrieved from http://www.americantelemed.org/docs/default-source/standards/practice-guidelines-for-videoconferencing-based-telemental-health.pdf?sfvrsn=6

American Telemedicine Association. (2010). *A blueprint for telerehabilitation guidelines.* Retrieved from: http://www.americantelemed.org/resources/telemedicine-practice-guidelines/telemedicine-practice-guidelines/blueprint-for-telerehabilitation-guidelines#.VLGQQivF98E

American Telemedicine Association. (2014). *State telemedicine legislation tracking.* Retrieved from http://www.americantelemed.org/docs/default-source/policy/2014-ata-state-legislation-matrixBD6205D8982E.pdf

American Telemedicine Association Telepresenting Standards and Guidelines Working Group. (2011). *Expert consensus recommendations for videoconferencing-based telepresenting.* Retrieved from http://www.americantelemed.org/resources/standards/ata-standards-guidelines/recommendations-for-videoconferencing-based-telepresenting#.U-rVffldWSo

Andersson, G., & Cuijpers, P. (2009). Internet-based and other computerized psychological treatments for adult depression: A meta-analysis. *Cognitive Behaviour Therapy, 38*, 196–205. http://dx.doi.org/10.1080/16506070903318960

Arora, S., Thornton, K., Komaromy, M., Kalishman, S., Katzman, J., & Duhigg, D. (2014). Demonopolizing medical knowledge. *Academic Medicine, 89*, 30–32. http://dx.doi.org/10.1097/ACM.0000000000000051

Arora, S., Thornton, K., Murata, G., Deming, P., Kalishman, S., Dion, D., . . . Qualls, C. (2011). Outcomes of treatment for hepatitis C virus infection by primary care providers. *The New England Journal of Medicine, 364*, 2199–2207. http://dx.doi.org/10.1056/NEJMoa1009370

Backhaus, A., Agha, Z., Maglione, M. L., Repp, A., Ross, B., Zuest, D., . . . Thorp, S. R. (2012). Videoconferencing psychotherapy: A systematic review. *Psychological Services, 9*, 111–131. http://dx.doi.org/10.1037/a0027924

Barnett, J. E., Kelly, J. F., & Roberts, M. C. (Eds.). (2011). Telehealth and technology innovation in professional psychology [Special issue]. *Professional Psychology: Research and Practice, 42*(6).

Barnett, J. E., & Molzon, C. H. (2014). Clinical supervision of psychotherapy: Essential ethics issues for supervisors and supervisees. *Journal of Clinical Psychology, 70*, 1051–1061. http://dx.doi.org/10.1002/jclp.22126

Bartram, D. (2006). Testing on the Internet: Issues, challenges and opportunities in the field of occupational assessment. In D. Bartram & R. K. Hambelton (Eds.), *Computer-based testing and the Internet: Issues and advances* (pp. 13–37). Hoboken, NJ: Wiley.

Batastini, A. B., McDonald, B. R., & Morgan, R. D. (2012). Videoconferencing in forensic and correctional practice. In K. Myers & C. Turvey (Eds.), *Telemental health: Clinical, technical and administrative foundations for evidence-based practice* (pp. 251–271). New York, NY: Elsevier.

Bennett, K., McElroy, J. A., Johnson, A. O., Munk, N., & Everett, K. D. (2015, March). A persistent disparity: Smoking in rural sexual and gender minorities. *LGBT Health, 2*, 62–70.

Benton, S. A., Snowden, S., Heesacker, M., & Lee, G. A. (2015, August). *Efficacy of low intensity–high engagement online therapy for anxiety in college students.* Poster session presented at the American Psychological Association Annual Convention, Toronto, Ontario, Canada.

Bower, P., & Gilbody, S. (2005). Stepped care in psychological therapies: Access, effectiveness and efficiency (Narrative literature review). *British Journal of Psychiatry, 186*, 11–17. http://dx.doi.org/10.1192/bjp.186.1.11

Brooks, E., Novins, D. K., Noe, T., Bair, B., Dailey, N., Lowe, J., . . . Shore, J. H. (2013). Reaching rural communities with culturally appropriate care: A model for adapting remote monitoring to American Indian veterans with posttraumatic stress disorder. *Telemedicine and e-Health, 19*, 272–277. http://dx.doi.org/10.1089/tmj.2012.0117

Brooks, E., Spargo, G., Yellowlees, P., O'Neill, P., & Shore, J. H. (2012). Integrating culturally appropriate care into telemental health practice. In K. Myers & C. Turvey (Eds.), *Telemental health: Clinical, technical and administrative foundations for evidence-based practice* (pp. 63–82). New York, NY: Elsevier.

Buchanan, T., Johnson, J. A., & Goldberg, L. R. (2005). Implementing a five-factor personality inventory for use on the Internet. *European Journal of Psychological Assessment, 21*, 116–128. http://dx.doi.org/10.1027/1015-5759.21.2.115

Burns, M. N., Begale, M., Duffecy, J., Gergle, D., Karr, C. J., Giangrande, E., & Mohr, D. C. (2011). Harnessing context sensing to develop a mobile intervention for depression. *Journal of Medical Internet Research, 13*(3), e55. http://dx.doi.org/10.2196/jmir.1838

Cain, S., Nelson, E.-L., & Myers, K. (2015). Telepsychiatry. In M. K. Dulcan (Ed.), *Dulcan's textbook of child and adolescent psychiatry.* Washington, DC: American Psychiatric Publishing.

California Telehealth Resource Center. (2014). *The CTRC Telehealth Program Developer kit.* Retrieved from http://www.telehealthresourcecenter.org/sites/main/files/file-attachments/complete-program-developer-kit-2014-web1.pdf

Callan, J., Maheu, M., & Bucky, S. (in press). Crisis in the behavioral health classroom: Enhancing knowledge, skills, and attitudes in telehealth training. In M. Maheu, K. Drude, & S. Wright (Eds.), *Field guide to evidence-based, technology careers in behavioral health: Professional opportunities for the 21st century.* New York, NY: Springer.

Casavant, D. W., McManus, M. L., Parsons, S. K., Zurakowski, D., & Graham, R. J. (2014). Trial of telemedicine for patients on home ventilator support: Feasibility, confidence in clinical management and use in medical decision-making. *Journal of Telemedicine and Telecare, 20,* 441–449. http://dx.doi.org/10.1177/1357633X14555620

Chakravarty, S., Cantor, J. C., Walkup, J., & Tong, J. (2014). *The role of behavioral health conditions in avoidable hospital use and cost.* New Brunswick, NJ: Rutgers Center for State Health Policy.

Chen, M. (2002). Leveraging the asymmetric sensitivity of eye contact for videoconferencing. In L. Terveen (Ed.), *Proceedings of the SIGCHI Conference on Human Factors in Computing Systems* (pp. 49–56). Minneapolis, MN: ACM Press.

Chi, N. C., & Demiris, G. (2015). A systematic review of telehealth tools and interventions to support family caregivers. *Journal of Telemedicine and Telecare, 21,* 37–44.

Chong, J., & Moreno, F. (2012). Feasibility and acceptability of clinic-based telepsychiatry for low-income Hispanic primary care patients. *Telemedicine and e-Health, 18,* 297–304. http://dx.doi.org/10.1089/tmj.2011.0126

Colbow, A. J. (2013). Looking to the future: Integrating telemental health therapy into psychologist training. *Training and Education in Professional Psychology, 7,* 155–165. http://dx.doi.org/10.1037/a0033454

Cuijpers, P., Marks, I. M., van Straten, A., Cavanagh, K., Gega, L., & Andersson, G. (2009). Computer-aided psychotherapy for anxiety disorders: A meta-analytic review. *Cognitive Behaviour Therapy, 38,* 66–82. http://dx.doi.org/10.1080/16506070802694776

Cunningham, P. J. (2009). Beyond parity: Primary care physicians' perspectives on access to mental health care. *Health Affairs, 28,* w490–w501. http://dx.doi.org/10.1377/hlthaff.28.3.w490

Duncan, A., Nelson, E.-L., Maheu, M., Glueckauf, R., Drude, K., & Gustafson, D. (2013, November). *Technology training in psychology internships.* Poster presented at the Association of Behavioral and Cognitive Therapies annual convention, Nashville, TN.

Duncan, A., Velasquez, S., & Nelson, E.-L. (2014). Using videoconferencing to provide psychological services to rural children and adolescents: A review and case example [Special section]. *Journal of Clinical Child and Adolescent Psychology, 43,* 115–127. http://dx.doi.org/10.1080/15374416.2013.836452

Dunstan, D. A., & Tooth, S. M. (2012). Treatment via videoconferencing: A pilot study of delivery by clinical psychology trainees. *Australian Journal of Rural Health, 20,* 88–94.

Earnshaw, V. A., Bogart, L. M., Dovidio, J. F., & Williams, D. R. (2013). Stigma and racial/ethnic HIV disparities: Moving toward resilience. *American Psychologist, 68,* 225–236. http://dx.doi.org/10.1037/a0032705

Falender, C. A., Shafranske, E. P., & Falicov, C. J. (Eds.). (2014). *Multiculturalism and diversity in clinical supervision: A competency-based approach.* Washington, DC: American Psychological Association.

Federation of State Medical Boards. (2013). *Telemedicine overview: Board-by-board approach.* Retrieved from http://www.fsmb.org

Forducey, P. G., Glueckauf, R. L., Bergquist, T. F., Maheu, M. M., & Yutsis, M. (2012). Telehealth for persons with severe functional disabilities and their caregivers: Facilitating self-care management in the home setting. *Psychological Services, 9,* 144–162. http://dx.doi.org/10.1037/a0028112

Fortney, J. C., Pyne, J. M., Kimbrell, T. A., Hudson, T. J., Robinson, D. E., Schneider, R., . . . Schnurr, P. P. (2015). Telemedicine-based collaborative care for posttraumatic stress disorder: A randomized clinical trial. *JAMA Psychiatry, 72,* 58–67.

Glueckauf, R. L., Davis, W. S., Willis, F., Sharma, D., Gustafson, D. J., Hayes, J., . . . Springer, J. (2012). Telephone-based, cognitive-behavioral therapy for African American dementia caregivers with depression: Initial findings. *Rehabilitation Psychology, 57,* 124–139.

Goldstein, F., & Myers, K. (2014). Telemental health: A new collaboration for pediatricians and child psychiatrists. *Pediatric Annals, 43,* 79–84. http://dx.doi.org/10.3928/00904481-20140127-12

Grady, B., Myers, K. M., Nelson, E.-L., Belz, N., Bennett, L., Carnahan, L., . . . Voyles, D. (2011). Evidence-based practice for telemental health. *Telemedicine and e-Health, 17,* 131–148. http://dx.doi.org/10.1089/tmj.2010.0158

Grayson, D. M., & Monk, A. F. (2003). Are you looking at me? Eye contact and desktop video conferencing. *ACM Transactions on Computer-Human Interaction, 10,* 221–243. http://dx.doi.org/10.1145/937549.937552

Gros, D. F., Morland, L. A., Greene, C. J., Acierno, R., Strachan, M., Egede, L. E., . . . Frueh, C. (2013). Delivery of evidence-based psychotherapy via video telehealth. *Journal of Psychopathology and Behavioral Assessment, 35*, 506–521. http://dx.doi.org/10.1007/s10862-013-9363-4

Gros, D. F., Veronee, K., Strachan, M., Ruggiero, K. J., & Acierno, R. (2011). Managing suicidality in home-based telehealth. *Journal of Telemedicine and Telecare, 17*, 332–335. http://dx.doi.org/10.1258/jtt.2011.101207

Gupta, A., & Sao, D. (2011). The constitutionality of current legal barriers to telemedicine in the United States: Analysis and future directions of its relationship to national and international health care reform. *Health Matrix, 21*, 385–442.

Hassija, C., & Gray, M. J. (2011). The effectiveness and feasibility of videoconferencing technology to provide evidence-based treatment to rural domestic violence and sexual assault populations. *Telemedicine and e-Health, 17*, 309–315. http://dx.doi.org/10.1089/tmj.2010.0147

Health Resources and Services Administration. (2010). *Health licensing board report to Congress.* Retrieved from http://docplayer.net/131532-Health-licensing-board-report-to-congress.html

Health Resources and Services Administration. (2014). *Shortage designation: Health professional shortage areas & medically underserved areas/populations.* Retrieved from http://www.hrsa.gov/shortage/

Hilgart, J. S., Hayward, J. A., Coles, B., & Iredale, R. (2012). Telegenetics: A systematic review of telemedicine in genetics services. *Genetics in Medicine, 14*, 765–776. http://dx.doi.org/10.1038/gim.2012.40

Hilty, D. M., Ferrer, D. C., Parish, M. B., Johnston, B., Callahan, E. J., & Yellowlees, P. M. (2013). The effectiveness of telemental health: A 2013 review. *Telemedicine and e-Health, 19*, 444–454. http://dx.doi.org/10.1089/tmj.2013.0075

Hook, J. N., Davis, D. E., Owen, J., Worthington, E. L., Jr., & Utsey, S. O. (2013). Cultural humility: Measuring openness to culturally diverse clients. *Journal of Counseling Psychology, 60*, 353–366. http://dx.doi.org/10.1037/a0032595

IHS. (2014). *Telehealth report.* Retrieved from http://eecatalog.com/medical/files/2014/01/IHS-Top-Healthcare-Technology-Trend-Predictions-for-2014.pdf

Institute of Medicine. (2001). *Crossing the quality chasm: A new health system for the 21st century.* Washington, DC: National Academies Press.

Joinson, A. (1999). Social desirability, anonymity, and internet-based questionnaires. *Behavior Research Methods, Instruments, & Computers, 31*, 433–438. http://dx.doi.org/10.3758/BF03200723

Keynejad, R., Ali, F. R., Finlayson, A. E., Handuleh, J., Adam, G., Bowen, J. S., . . . Whitwell, S. (2013). Telemedicine for peer-to-peer psychiatry learning between U.K. and Somaliland medical students. *Academic Psychiatry, 37*, 182–186. http://dx.doi.org/10.1176/appi.ap.11080148

Kim, H. S., & Jeong, H. S. (2007). A nurse short message service by cellular phone in type-2 diabetic patients for six months. *Journal of Clinical Nursing, 16*, 1082–1087. http://dx.doi.org/10.1111/j.1365-2702.2007.01698.x

Kim, H., Spaulding, R., Werkowitch, M., Yadrich, D., Pimjariyakul, U., Gilroy, R., & Smith, C. E. (2014). Costs of multidisciplinary parenteral nutrition care provided at a distance via mobile tablets. *Journal of Parenteral and Enteral Nutrition, 38*(Suppl. 2), 50S–57S. http://dx.doi.org/10.1177/0148607114550692

Knapp, S., Younggren, J. N., VandeCreek, L., Harris, E., & Martin, J. N. (2013). *Assessing and managing risk in psychological practice: An individualized approach* (2nd ed.). Washington, DC: The Trust.

Kneebone, E., & Berube, A. (2014). *Confronting suburban poverty in America.* Washington, DC: Brookings Institution.

Kobak, K. A., Craske, M. G., Rose, R. D., & Wolitsky-Taylor, K. (2013). Web-based therapist training on cognitive behavior therapy for anxiety disorders: A pilot study. *Psychotherapy, 50*, 235–247. http://dx.doi.org/10.1037/a0030568

Kongsved, S. M., Basnov, M., Holm-Christensen, K., & Hjollund, N. H. (2007). Response rate and completeness of questionnaires: A randomized study of Internet versus paper-and-pencil versions. *Journal of Medical Internet Research, 9*(3), e25. http://dx.doi.org/10.2196/jmir.9.3.e25

Kramer, G. M., & Luxton, D. D. (2015). Telemental health for children and adolescents: An overview of legal, regulatory, and risk management issues. *Journal of Child and Adolescent Psychopharmacology.* Advance online publication. http://dx.doi.org/10.1089/cap.2015.0018

Kramer, G. M., Mishkind, M. C., Luxton, D. D., & Shore, J. H. (2013). Managing risk and protecting privacy in telemental health: An overview of legal, regulatory, and risk management issues. In K. Myers & C. L. Turvey (Eds.), *Telemental health: Clinical, technical and administrative foundations for evidence-based practice* (pp. 83–107). Waltham, MA: Elsevier.

Kubota, A., Fujita, M., & Hatano, Y. (2004). Development and effects of a health promotion program utilizing the mail function of mobile phones. *Japanese Journal of Public Health, 51*, 862–873.

L'Abate, L. (2013). *Clinical psychology and psychotherapy as a science: An iconoclastic perspective.* New York, NY: Springer-Science. http://dx.doi.org/10.1007/978-1-4614-4451-0

Larson, J. E., & Corrigan, P. W. (2010). Psychotherapy for self-stigma among rural clients. *Journal of Clinical Psychology, 66*, 524–536.

León, A., Cáceres, C., Fernández, E., Chausa, P., Martin, M., Codina, C., . . . García, F. (2011). A new multidisciplinary home care telemedicine system to monitor stable chronic human immunodeficiency virus-infected patients: A randomized study. *PLoS ONE, 6*, e14515. http://dx.doi.org/10.1371/journal.pone.0014515

Lopez, M. H., Gonzalez-Barrera, A., & Patten, E. (2013). *Closing the digital divide: Latinos and technology adoption.* Washington, DC: Pew Hispanic Center. Retrieved from http://www.pewhispanic.org/2013/03/07/closing-the-digital-divide-latinos-and-technology-adoption/

Lupton, D. (2013). Quantifying the body: Monitoring and measuring health in the age of mHealth technologies. *Critical Public Health, 23,* 393–403. http://dx.doi.org/10.1080/09581596.2013.794931

Lutwak, N., & Dill, C. (2013). An innovative method to deliver treatment of military sexual trauma and post-traumatic stress disorder. *Military Medicine, 178,* 1039–1040. http://dx.doi.org/10.7205/MILMED-D-13-00226

Luxton, D. D. (2013). Considerations for planning and evaluating economic analyses of telemental health. *Psychological Services, 10,* 276–282. http://dx.doi.org/10.1037/a0030658

Luxton, D. D. (2014a). Artificial intelligence in psychological practice: Current and future applications and implications. *Professional Psychology: Research and Practice, 45,* 332–339. http://dx.doi.org/10.1037/a0034559

Luxton, D. D. (2014b). Recommendations for the ethical use and design of artificial intelligent care providers. *Artificial Intelligence in Medicine, 62,* 1–10. doi:10.1016/j.artmed.2014.06.004

Luxton, D. D. (Ed.). (2015). *Artificial intelligence in behavioral and mental health care.* New York, NY: Elsevier/Academic Press. http://dx.doi.org/10.1016/B978-0-12-420248-1.00001-5

Luxton, D. D., Hansen, R. N., & Stanfill, K. (2014). Mobile app self-care versus in-office care for stress reduction: A cost minimization analysis. *Journal of Telemedicine and Telecare, 20,* 431–435. http://dx.doi.org/10.1177/1357633X14555616

Luxton, D. D., June, J. D., & Chalker, S. (2015). Mobile health technologies for suicide prevention: Feature review and recommendations for use in clinical care. *Current Treatment Options in Psychiatry, 2,* 349–362. http://dx.doi.org/10.1007/s40501-015-0057-2

Luxton, D. D., Kayl, R. A., & Mishkind, M. C. (2012). mHealth data security: The need for HIPAA-compliant standardization. *Telemedicine and e-Health, 18,* 284–288. http://dx.doi.org/10.1089/tmj.2011.0180

Luxton, D. D., McCann, R. A., Bush, N. E., Mishkind, M. C., & Reger, G. M. (2011). mHealth for mental health: Integrating smartphone technology in behavioral healthcare. *Professional Psychology: Research and Practice, 42,* 505–512. http://dx.doi.org/10.1037/a0024485

Luxton, D. D., Mishkind, M. C., Crumpton, R. M., Ayers, T. D., & Mysliwiec, V. (2012). Usability and feasibility of smartphone video capabilities for telehealth care in the U.S. military. *Telemedicine and e-Health, 18,* 409–412. http://dx.doi.org/10.1089/tmj.2011.0219

Luxton, D. D., O'Brien, K., McCann, R. A., & Mishkind, M. C. (2012). Home-based telemental healthcare safety planning: What you need to know. *Telemedicine and e-Health, 18*, 629–633. http://dx.doi.org/10.1089/tmj.2012.0004

Luxton, D. D., O'Brien, K., Pruitt, L. D., Johnson, K., & Kramer, G. (2014). Suicide risk management during clinical telepractice. *International Journal of Psychiatry in Medicine, 48*, 19–31. http://dx.doi.org/10.2190/PM.48.1.c

Luxton, D. D., Pruitt, L. D., & Osenbach, J. E. (2014). Best practices for remote psychological assessment via telehealth technologies. *Professional Psychology: Research and Practice, 45*, 27–35. http://dx.doi.org/10.1037/a0034547

Luxton, D. D., Sirotin, A. P., & Mishkind, M. C. (2010). Safety of telemental healthcare delivered to clinically unsupervised settings: A systematic review. *Telemedicine and e-Health, 16*, 705–711. http://dx.doi.org/10.1089/tmj.2009.0179

Maheu, M. M. (2003). The online clinical practice management model. *Psychotherapy: Theory, Research, Practice, Training, 40*, 20–32. http://dx.doi.org/10.1037/0033-3204.40.1-2.20

Maheu, M., Drude, K., & Wright, S. (Eds.) (2015). *Field guide to evidence-based, technology careers in behavioral health: Professional career opportunities for the 21st century.* New York, NY: Springer.

Maheu, M. M., & Gordon, B. L. (2000). Counseling and therapy on the Internet: Legal, ethical and practice issues [Special section]. *Professional Psychology: Research and Practice, 31*, 484–489. http://dx.doi.org/10.1037/0735-7028.31.5.484

Maheu, M., & McMenamin, J. (2004). Successful website construction and management: Harnessing the skill and enthusiasm of volunteers. In P. Whitten & D. Cook (Eds.), *Understanding health communication technologies* (pp. 187–192). San Francisco, CA: Jossey-Bass.

Maheu, M. M., & McMenamin, J. (2013, March 28). Telepsychiatry: The perils of using Skype. *Psychiatric Times.* Retrieved from http://www.psychiatrictimes.com/display/article/10168/2131095

Maheu, M., Pulier, M., McMenamin, J., & Posen, L. (2012). The future of telepsychology, telehealth, and various technologies in psychological research. *Professional Psychology: Research and Practice, 43*, 613–621. http://dx.doi.org/10.1037/a0029458

Maheu, M. M., Pulier, M. L., & Roy, S. (2013). Finding, evaluating, and using smartphone applications. In G. P. Koocher, J. C. Norcross, & B. A. Greene (Eds.), *Psychologists' desk reference* (3rd ed., pp. 705–708). New York, NY: Oxford University Press. http://dx.doi.org/10.1093/med:psych/9780199845491.003.0136

Maheu, M. M., Pulier, M. L., Wilhelm, F. H., McMenamin, J., & Brown-Connolly, N. (2004). *The mental health professional and the new technologies: A handbook for practice today.* Mahwah, NJ: Erlbaum.

Maheu, M., Whitten, P., & Allen, A. (2001). *E-health, telehealth, and telemedicine: A guide to start-up and success.* San Francisco, CA: Jossey-Bass.

McClellan, F., Washington, M., Ruff, R., & Selkirk, S. M. (2013). Early and innovative symptomatic care to improve quality of life of ALS patients at Cleveland VA ALS Center. *Journal of Rehabilitation Research and Development, 50*(4), vii–xvi. http://dx.doi.org/10.1682/JRRD.2013.05.0107

Merikangas, K. R., He, J. P., Burstein, M., Swanson, S. A., Avenevoli, S., Cui, L., . . . Swendsen, J. (2010). Lifetime prevalence of mental disorders in U.S. adolescents: Results from the National Comorbidity Survey Replication—Adolescent Supplement (NCS-A). *Journal of the American Academy of Child & Adolescent Psychiatry, 49,* 980–989. http://dx.doi.org/10.1016/j.jaac.2010.05.017

Merikangas, K. R., He, J. P., Burstein, M., Swendsen, J., Avenevoli, S., Case, B., . . . Olfson, M. (2011). Service utilization for lifetime mental disorders in U.S. adolescents: Results of the National Comorbidity Survey-Adolescent Supplement (NCS-A). *Journal of the American Academy of Child & Adolescent Psychiatry, 50,* 32–45. http://dx.doi.org/10.1016/j.jaac.2010.10.006

Miyamoto, S., Dharmar, M., Boyle, C., Yang, N. H., MacLeod, K., Rogers, K., . . . Marcin, J. P. (2014). Impact of telemedicine on the quality of forensic sexual abuse examinations in rural communities. *Child Abuse & Neglect, 38,* 1533–1539. http://dx.doi.org/10.1016/j.chiabu.2014.04.015

Mohr, D. C., Burns, M. N., Schueller, S. M., Clarke, G., & Klinkman, M. (2013). Behavioral intervention technologies: Evidence review and recommendations for future research in mental health. *General Hospital Psychiatry, 35,* 332–338. http://dx.doi.org/10.1016/j.genhosppsych.2013.03.008

Mohr, D. C., Vella, L., Hart, S., Heckman, T., & Simon, G. (2008). The effect of telephone-administered psychotherapy on symptoms of depression and attrition: A meta-analysis. *Clinical Psychology: Science and Practice, 15,* 243–253. http://dx.doi.org/10.1111/j.1468-2850.2008.00134.x

Myers, K., Cain, S., & Work Group on Quality Issues. (2008). Practice parameter for telepsychiatry with children and adolescents. *Journal of the American Academy of Child & Adolescent Psychiatry, 47,* 1468–1483. http://dx.doi.org/10.1097/CHI.0b013e31818b4e13

Myers, K. M., & Lieberman, D. (2013). Telemental health: Responding to mandates for reform in primary healthcare. *Telemedicine and e-Health, 19,* 438–443. http://dx.doi.org/10.1089/tmj.2013.0084

Myers, K., & Turvey, C. (Eds.). (2012). *Telemental health: Clinical, technical and administrative foundations for evidence-based practice.* New York, NY: Elsevier.

National Association of Social Workers. (2008). *Code of ethics of the National Association of Social Workers.* Retrieved from http://www.socialworkers.org/pubs/code/code.asp

National Institute of Mental Health. (n.d.). *Statistics: Any disorder among adults.* Retrieved from http://www.nimh.nih.gov/statistics/1ANYDIS_ADULT.shtml

Nelson, E.-L., & Bui, T. (2010). Rural telepsychology services for children and adolescents. *Journal of Clinical Psychology, 66*, 490–501.

Nelson, E.-L., Bui, T., & Sharp, S. (2011). Telemental health competencies: Training examples from a youth depression telemedicine clinic. In M. Gregerson (Ed.), *Technology innovations for behavioral education* (pp. 41–47). New York, NY: Springer. http://dx.doi.org/10.1007/978-1-4419-9392-2_5

Nelson, E.-L., Davis, K., & Velasquez, S. E. (2012). Telemedicine and ethics. In K. Myers & C. Turvey (Eds.), *Telemental health: Clinical, technical and administrative foundations for evidence-based practice* (pp. 47–52). New York, NY: Elsevier.

Nelson, E.-L., & Duncan, A. B. (2015). Cognitive behavioral therapy using televideo. *Cognitive and Behavioral Practice, 22*, 269–280.

Nelson, E.-L., Mulhern, M., Bush, C., & Groneman, B. (2011). Televideo support services for rural cancer patients and their families [Abstract]. *Telemedicine and e-Health, 17*(4).

Nelson, E.-L., & Patton, S. (in press). Telepsychology update. *Journal of Child and Adolescent Psychopharmacology.*

Nelson, E.-L., & Velasquez, S. E. (2011). Implementing psychological services over televideo. *Professional Psychology: Research and Practice, 42*, 535–542. http://dx.doi.org/10.1037/a0026178

Ohio Psychological Association. (2013). *Areas of competence for psychologists in telepsychology.* Retrieved from http://www.ohpsych.org/about/files/2012/03/FINAL_COMPETENCY_DRAFT.pdf

Oliver, D. P., Demiris, G., Wittenberg-Lyles, E., Washington, K., Day, T., & Novak, H. (2012). A systematic review of the evidence base for telehospice. *Telemedicine and e-Health, 18*, 38–47. http://dx.doi.org/10.1089/tmj.2011.0061

Pabian, Y. L., Welfel, E., & Beebe, R. S. (2009). Psychologists' knowledge of their state laws pertaining to Tarasoff-type situations. *Professional Psychology: Research and Practice, 40*, 8–14. http://dx.doi.org/10.1037/a0014784

Pruitt, L. D., Luxton, D. D., & Shore, P. (2014). Additional clinical benefits of home-based telemental health. *Professional Psychology: Research and Practice, 45*, 340–346. http://dx.doi.org/10.1037/a0035461

Reese, R. J., Aldarondo, F., Anderson, C. R., Lee, S. J., Miller, T. W., & Burton, D. (2009). Telehealth in clinical supervision: A comparison of supervision formats. *Journal of Telemedicine and Telecare, 15*, 356–361. http://dx.doi.org/10.1258/jtt.2009.090401

Reese, R. M., Braun, M. J., Hoffmeier, S., Stickle, L., Rinner, L., Smith, C., . . . Hadorn, M. (2015). Primary evidence for the integrated systems using telemedicine. *Telemedicine and e-Health, 21*, 581–587.

Reips, U.-D. (2000). The web experiment method: Advantages, disadvantages, and solutions. In M. H. Birnbaum (Ed.), *Psychological experiments on the Internet* (pp. 89–117). San Diego, CA: Academic Press.

Richards, D. A., Bower, P., Pagel, C., Weaver, A., Utley, M., Cape, J., . . . Vasilakis, C. (2012). Delivering stepped care: An analysis of implementation in routine practice. *Implementation Science, 7*, 3. http://dx.doi.org/10.1186/1748-5908-7-3

Ritterband, L. M., Gonder-Frederick, L. A., Cox, D. J., Clifton, A. D., West, R. W., & Borowitz, S. M. (2003). Internet interventions: In review, in use, and into the future. *Professional Psychology: Research & Practice, 34*, 527–534.

Rousmaniere, T., Abbass, A., & Frederickson, J. (2014). New developments in technology-assisted supervision and training: A practical overview. *Journal of Clinical Psychology, 70*, 1082–1093. http://dx.doi.org/10.1002/jclp.22129

Rousmaniere, T., Abbass, A., Frederickson, J., Henning, I., & Taubner, S. (2014). Videoconference for psychotherapy training and supervision: Two case examples. *American Journal of Psychotherapy, 68*, 231–250.

Saberi, P., Yuan, P., John, M., Sheon, N., & Johnson, M. O. (2013). A pilot study to engage and counsel HIV-positive African American youth via telehealth technology. *AIDS Patient Care and STDs, 27*, 529–532. http://dx.doi.org/10.1089/apc.2013.0185

Saifu, H. N., Asch, S. M., Goetz, M. B., Smith, J. P., Graber, C. J., Schaberg, D., & Sun, B. C. (2012). Evaluation of human immunodeficiency virus and hepatitis C telemedicine clinics. *The American Journal of Managed Care, 18*, 207–212.

Santiago-Rivera, A. L., Arredondo, P., & Gallardo-Cooper, M. (2002). *Counseling Latinos and la familia: A practical guide.* Thousand Oaks, CA: Sage.

Shore, J. H., Bloom, J. D., Manson, S. M., & Whitener, R. J. (2008). Telepsychiatry with rural American Indians: Issues in civil commitments. *Behavioral Sciences & the Law, 26*, 287–300. http://dx.doi.org/10.1002/bsl.813

Shore, J., Kaufmann, L. J., Brooks, E., Bair, B. D., Dailey, N., Richardson, W. J. B., . . . Manson, S. (2012). Review of American Indian veteran telemental health. *Telemedicine and e-Health, 18*, 87–94.

Shore, J. H., & Manson, S. M. (2005). A developmental model for rural telepsychiatry. *Psychiatric Services, 56*, 976–980. http://dx.doi.org/10.1176/appi.ps.56.8.976

Shore, J. H., Mishkind, M. C., Bernard, J., Doarn, C. R., Bell, I., Jr., Bhatla, R., . . . Vo, A. (2014). A lexicon of assessment and outcome measures for telemental health. *Telemedicine and e-Health, 20*, 282–292. http://dx.doi.org/10.1089/tmj.2013.0357

Shore, J. H., Savin, D. M., Novins, D., & Manson, S. M. (2006). Cultural aspects of telepsychiatry. *Journal of Telemedicine and Telecare, 12*, 116–121. http://dx.doi.org/10.1258/135763306776738602

Slone, N. C., Reese, R. J., & McClellan, M. J. (2012). Telepsychology outcome research with children and adolescents: A review of the literature. *Psychological Services, 9*, 272–292. http://dx.doi.org/10.1037/a0027607

Smalley, B., Warren, J., & Rainer, J. (2012). *Rural mental health: Issues, policies, and best practices.* New York, NY: Springer.

Smith, A. (2014a, January). *African Americans and technology use* (Pew Research Center report). Retrieved from http://www.pewinternet.org/2014/01/06/african-americans-and-technology-use/

Smith, A. (2014b, April). *Older adults and technology use* (Pew Research Center report). Retrieved from http://www.pewinternet.org/2014/04/03/older-adults-and-technology-use/

Spaulding, R., Cain, S., & Sonnenschein, K. (2011). Urban telepsychiatry: Uncommon service for a common need. *Child and Adolescent Psychiatric Clinics of North America, 20*, 29–39. http://dx.doi.org/10.1016/j.chc.2010.08.010

Strachan, M., Gros, D. F., Yuen, E., Ruggiero, K. J., Foa, E. B., & Acierno, R. (2012). Home-based telehealth to deliver evidence-based psychotherapy in veterans with PTSD. *Contemporary Clinical Trials, 33*, 402–409. http://dx.doi.org/10.1016/j.cct.2011.11.007

Szeftel, R., Mandelbaum, S., Sulman-Smith, H., Naqvi, S., Lawrence, L., Szeftel, Z., . . . Gross, L. (2011). Telepsychiatry for children with developmental disabilities: Applications for patient care and medical education. *Child and Adolescent Psychiatric Clinics of North America, 20*, 95–111. http://dx.doi.org/10.1016/j.chc.2010.08.011

Tam, T., Cafazzo, J. A., Seto, E., Salenieks, M. E., & Rossos, P. G. (2007). Perception of eye contact in video teleconsultation. *Journal of Telemedicine and Telecare, 13*, 35–39. http://dx.doi.org/10.1258/135763307779701239

Telehealth Services. (2011). 42 CFR 410.78. Retrieved from http://www.gpo.gov/fdsys/granule/CFR-2011-title42-vol2/CFR-2011-title42-vol2-sec410-78

Thomas, L., & Capistrant, G. (2015). *State telemedicine gaps analysis.* Retrieved from http://www.americantelemed.org/policy/state-policy-resource-center#.VbEuHKFlC71

Tousignant, M., Corriveau, H., Kairy, D., Berg, K., Dubois, M. F., Gosselin, S., . . . Danells, C. (2014). Tai Chi-based exercise program provided via telerehabilitation compared to home visits in a post-stroke population who have returned home without intensive rehabilitation: Study protocol for a randomized, non-inferiority clinical trial. *Trials*, *15*, 42. http://dx.doi.org/10.1186/1745-6215-15-42

Turvey, C., Coleman, M., Dennison, O., Drude, K., Goldenson, M., Hirsch, P., . . . Bernard, J. (2013). ATA practice guidelines for video-based online mental health services. *Telemedicine and e-Health*, *19*, 722–730. http://dx.doi.org/10.1089/tmj.2013.9989

Turvey, C. L., Willyard, D., Hickman, D. H., Klein, D. M., & Kukoyi, O. (2007). Telehealth screen for depression in a chronic illness care management program. *Telemedicine and e-Health*, *13*, 51–56. http://dx.doi.org/10.1089/tmj.2006.0036

U.S. Department of Health and Human Services, Substance Abuse and Mental Health Services Administration. (2013a). *Behavioral Health, United States, 2012* (HHS Publication No. (SMA) 13-4797). Rockville, MD: Author.

U.S. Department of Health and Human Services, Substance Abuse and Mental Health Services Administration. (2013b). *Report to Congress on the nation's substance abuse and mental health workforce issues.* Retrieved from http://store.samhsa.gov/shin/content//PEP13-RTC-BHWORK/PEP13-RTC-BHWORK.pdf

U.S. Department of Health and Human Services, Substance Abuse and Mental Health Services Administration, Center for Behavioral Health Statistics and Quality. (2012). *Results from the 2020 National Survey on Drug Use and Health: Mental health findings* (NSDUH Series H-42, HHS Publication No. (SMA) 11-4667). Rockville, MD: Author.

Weinstein, R. S., Lopez, A. M., Joseph, B. A., Erps, K. A., Holcomb, M., Barker, G. P., & Krupinski, E. A. (2014). Telemedicine, telehealth, and mobile health applications that work: Opportunities and barriers. *The American Journal of Medicine*, *127*, 183–187. http://dx.doi.org/10.1016/j.amjmed.2013.09.032

Wood, J., Miller, T. M., & Hargrove, D. S. (2005). Clinical supervision in rural settings: A telehealth model. *Professional Psychology: Research and Practice*, *36*, 173–179.

Ye, J., Shim, R., Lukaszewski, T., Yun, K., Kim, S. H., & Ruth, G. (2012). Telepsychiatry services for Korean immigrants. *Telemedicine and e-Health*, *18*, 797–802. doi:10.1089/tmj.2012.0041

Yellowlees, P. M., Odor, A., Iosif, A. M., Parish, M. B., Nafiz, N., Patrice, K., . . . Hilty, D. (2013). Transcultural psychiatry made simple—asynchronous telepsychiatry as an approach to providing culturally relevant care. *Telemedicine and e-Health*, *19*, 259–264. http://dx.doi.org/10.1089/tmj.2012.0077

Young, J. D., Patel, M., Badowski, M., Mackesy-Amiti, M. E., Vaughn, P., Shicker, L., . . . Ouellet, L. J. (2014). Improved virologic suppression with HIV subspecialty care in a large prison system using telemedicine: An observational study with historical controls. *Clinical Infectious Diseases*, *59*, 123–126. http://dx.doi.org/10.1093/cid/ciu222

Index

About the Authors

David D. Luxton, PhD, is CEO and founder of Luxton Labs LLC, a behavioral health technologies search and development company, chief science officer at NowMattersNow.org, and affiliate associate professor in the Department of Psychiatry and Behavioral Sciences at the University of Washington School of Medicine, Seattle. He previously served as a research health scientist at the Naval Health Research Center in San Diego, California, and as a research psychologist and program manager at the U.S. Army's National Center for Telehealth & Technology. Dr. Luxton's research and writing is focused in the areas of military and veterans' health, suicide prevention, telehealth, clinical best practices and ethics when using technology, and the study and development of emergent technologies in health care. He has served on numerous national workgroups and committees and is a highly sought after subject matter expert and consultant. Dr. Luxton is a licensed clinical psychologist and U.S. Air Force veteran.

Eve-Lynn Nelson, PhD, is a professor of pediatrics and telemedicine at the University of Kansas Medical Center (KUMC), where she directs the KU Center for Telemedicine and Telehealth. She also serves as the research liaison for the KU Institute for Community Engagement. Her research focuses on health services using telemedicine and videoconferencing technologies. She has served as principal investigator and collaborator on a number of grants pairing distance education and clinical telemedicine to address access gaps across the lifespan. Recent projects are the evaluation of mobile telebehavioral health approaches delivered to the home as well as a trial evaluating telebehavioral services to rural children living in poverty. In addition, Dr. Nelson spearheads KUMC's replication of the national Project Extension of Healthcare Outcomes. She is a licensed psychologist who leads a multidisciplinary telemedicine clinic providing services throughout rural and urban settings and across primary care clinics, schools, and other sites. She supervises health trainees across disciplines in learning about telemental health and adopting technologies into practice.

Marlene M. Maheu, PhD, is a consultant, trainer, author, and researcher. She is the executive director of the TeleMental Health Institute, Inc. For more than 20 years, Dr. Maheu's focus has been on the legal and ethical risk management issues related to the use of technologies in behavioral health. She has trained more than 15,000 licensed clinicians and overseen the development and delivery of professional training in telemental health via an eLearning platform that has served clinicians in 39 countries worldwide. She has written peer-reviewed articles, authored four telehealth textbooks, and served on professional association committees and task forces related to behavioral telehealth. Her vision and passion for the legal and ethical use of technology have led to her presidency of multiple nonprofit groups, including the American Counseling Association's Counseling and Technology Interest Network and the Coalition for Technology in Behavioral Science. In her consulting role, she has lead teams for elemental health program design and strategic planning, technology choices, technology development, staff recruitment, staff training, risk management, credentialing, reimbursement, and outcome research. Through a new company, BehaviorIT, she also consults with technology startup companies developing behavioral health technologies that seek to improve outcomes by automating behavioral services for employers, health plans, primary and specialty care offices, and universities.